Harvey Sag ....d in Medicine at
Oxford University and from 1984 worked as consultant
neur......... .. .. He
wa .... logy
at ... .arch
int... .. ..viou-
ra. .. .. a Movement and Memory
D........ Clinic, was a member of the Council of Management and Medical Advisory Panel of the Parkinson's Disease
Society, and is a member of various other bodies, including
the Association of British Neurologists, Corresponding Fel-
low of the American Academy of Neurology and the
European Society of Neurology.

He is now Professor Emeritus of Clinical Neurology and
works in private practice at Thornbury Hospital, Sheffield,
S10 3RR. He has founded the internet website
www.neuroconsult.co.uk which provides comprehensive
information on neurological disorders, including Parkinson's
disease.

The Parkinson's Disease Society is currently at 215 Vauxhall
Bridge Road, London SW1V 1EJ, telephone 020 7931 8080,
www.parkinsons.org.uk

PARKINSON'S DISEASE

*The essential guide
for sufferers and carers*

Professor Harvey Sagar

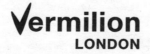
Vermilion
LONDON

First published by Macdonald Optima in 1991

1 3 5 7 9 10 8 6 4 2

This edition published in the United Kingdom in 2002
by Vermilion, an imprint of Ebury Press

Random House UK Ltd
Random House, 20 Vauxhall Bridge Road, London SW1V 2SA

Random House Australia (Pty) Ltd
20 Alfred Street, Milsons Point, Sydney
New South Wales 2016, Australia

Random House New Zealand Limited
18 Poland Road, Glenfield
Auckland 10 New Zealand

Random House South Africa (Pty) Limited
PO Box 337 Bergvlei South Africa

Random House UK Limited Reg. No. 954009

A CIP catalogue record for this book
is available from the British Library.

ISBN 0 09 188387 3

Typeset by Deltatype Ltd, Birkenhead, Merseyside

Printed and bound in Great Britain by
Mackays of Chatham, plc

Papers used by Vermilion are natural, recyclable products made
from wood grown in sustainable forests.

Contents

Preface

Over the last twenty years we have learnt an enormous amount about the problems of Parkinson's disease and its causes. Since the 1960s the treatment of Parkinson's disease has undergone almost revolutionary progress. The research effort that has been put into the condition over recent years is impressive and shows little sign of decreasing; each year seems to produce yet another exciting development. In the United Kingdom the Parkinson's Disease Society has continued to grow since its foundation in 1969 to provide a major input into research and welfare support for this condition. Of course, we do not yet know the true cause or have the definitive cure and, for many people, the disease still causes major difficulties in their ability to carry out tasks of everyday life. But the prospects for major steps forward in the treatment – or even prevention – of Parkinson's disease look better now than they ever have before.

Despite these thoughts the level of public awareness of Parkinson's disease is still remarkably low and misconceptions abound. Some people regard one brain disease as much like any other – a cause of unremitting loss of all physical and intellectual faculties over short periods of time. But for Parkinson's disease this is not the general truth. When I tell a patient for the first time that they have Parkinson's disease, I much more commonly have to correct pessimistic ideas that they have developed an untreatable fatal disease than to blunt their optimism and point out some of the potential problems that they have not appreciated. This book is partly written to correct this lack of awareness. In separate chapters we have described what Parkinson's disease is, what we know of its cause and ways in which it can be treated. We hope that the information will be sufficiently detailed for you to gain a much more balanced, up-to-date knowledge of the condition.

My work in a Movement Disorders Clinic shows me a broad spectrum of patients with Parkinson's disease and I am impressed how the condition affects people in such different ways. Although we tend to make generalizations when giving advice, it is important to realise that each patient is an individual. Not everyone has the same symptoms, or feels them to the same degree. Many people with Parkinson's disease are managing perfectly well but others do have persistent problems despite treatment, and sometimes severely. This book attempts to take account of these observations in several chapters on the symptoms of the disease. We have included a wide-ranging description of the problems of the condition, not because we believe that all patients are equally affected but because we wish to include advice on as many aspects of the disease as possible. In this way we hope to reach as many patients, relatives and interested people as we can.

The publishers would like to thank Jennie Smith for the illustrations, and Roche Products Ltd for the materials reproduced on pages 11, 12 and 41.

1

Why Parkinson's disease?

Parkinson's disease is named after an English doctor called James Parkinson who lived between 1755 and 1824. In 1817 he published a small book entitled *Essay on the Shaking Palsy* in which he described his own observations on six patients who had involuntary shaking of the arms, legs and body. James Parkinson recognized that the features of these six patients were all similar and differed from other medical causes of shaking that had been known up to that time. He called this new disease *paralysis agitans* (shaking palsy), but a French neurologist, Charcot, later suggested that the disease be named Parkinson's disease in honour of the man who first recognized it, and this term has remained ever since.

Interestingly, although James Parkinson is best known for his description of Parkinson's disease, he had many other interests. He wrote a number of articles for the medical journals on subjects as diverse as gout, appendicitis and the effects of being struck by lightning. He also wrote several books, including *The Villager's Friend and Physician, The Hospital Pupil* (about medical students) and *Hints for the Improvement of Trusses*. And his interests were not confined to medicine; he also wrote books on animal and vegetable fossils, which were accepted as key works in the scientific world at the time, and a compendium of chemistry called *The Chemical Pocket-Book*, which was as popular as his books on medicine and fossils. His most extraordinary activities, however, had nothing to do with medicine or science. Soon after the French Revolution, James Parkinson wrote a series of articles on political matters, and indeed was a keen political activist of the time. Britain was in a state of some political upheaval soon after the French Revolution, for many people saw unpleasant parallels between the inhumane and unjust government of France, which had just been overthrown, and that of Britain, which was still in power. For example, some areas of Britain, with very small populations, were sending as many MPs to Parliament as other areas with much larger populations. Accordingly, a number of reform societies were set up, devoted to the principle of political reform, and James Parkinson was a keen participant in these societies. His political articles were sometimes written in his own name, but were often written under a pen-name, Old Hubert; one such article against his staunchest political opponent was written in 1793 and called 'An Address to the Honorable Edmund Burke from the Swinish Multitude'. These political activities were no laughing matter; on one occasion, James Parkinson was summoned to give evidence regarding a plot to assassinate the King. It was fortunate for medicine that Parkinson himself was not on trial because conviction meant certain death, and it was not until 24 years later that he was to write his famous monograph on the shaking palsy!

James Parkinson's claims regarding his observations on the shaking palsy were very modest. In his monograph he introduces his findings with the statement that 'some ... explanation should be offered for the present publication: in which it is acknowledged that mere conjecture takes the place of experiment'. Nevertheless, 'to delay ... publication did not appear warrantable' because 'the disease had escaped particular notice'. James Parkinson went on to provide detailed descriptions of six patients, which have largely provided an accurate description of Parkinson's disease up to the present day.

Parkinson's disease and Parkinsonism

In this book, true Parkinson's disease, or *paralysis agitans*, as described by James Parkinson, will be referred to as idiopathic Parkinson's disease or simply Parkinson's disease.

James Parkinson recognized that there are other causes of tremor, apart from *paralysis agitans*, when he wrote 'Tremor can indeed only be considered a symptom, although several species of it must be admitted'. We now know that there are many conditions, some common and some rare, that look at first sight very much like Parkinson's disease, but which can usually be distinguished when a doctor carefully examines his patient. For example, patients who have had a number of small strokes may walk in a similar way to a patient with Parkinson's disease; and some forms of tremor run in families, although the afflicted members do not show the other problems, such as walking difficulty, that are experienced by many patients with Parkinson's disease.

Some diseases, however, are more like Parkinson's disease and may be difficult to distinguish, even by an experienced neurologist. These diseases are caused by problems with the nervous system quite distinct from those causing Parkinson's disease, and are clearly recognized by doctors as different diseases. Because these patients have problems that are like true Parkinson's disease, however, the term Parkinsonism is sometimes used to describe this sort of medical condition.

Conditions that may be confused with Parkinson's disease

- Benign essential tremor
- Infections
- Side-effects of drugs
- Poisonous substances
- Degenerative diseases of the nervous system
- Stroke
- Inherited diseases
- Head trauma
- Normal pressure hydrocephalus
- Thyroid disease and other similar metabolic disorders

Benign essential tremor

This condition causes shaking of the arms and the head; rarely, however, is there shaking of the legs, which, by contrast, are affected frequently in Parkinson's disease. The tremor is different from that of Parkinson's disease because it is usually a little faster and not quite so regular and rhythmic as the Parkinsonian tremor. Although it may be present at rest it is often made worse when the hands are used, such as in carrying cups of tea, and this may prove a great embarrassment as well as an inconvenience; writing is often a particular problem. In contrast, the tremor of Parkinson's disease is typically worse when the person is not using the limbs and, in most cases (although not all), the tremor improves when the limbs are used.

Benign essential tremor may develop at any age, from childhood to old age, but it is basically the same condition regardless of age of onset. It tends to get worse, but only over many years; indeed, patients have often had the tremor for very many years before they ever consult a doctor and even then because it has only just begun to cause real problems or embarrassment. This is why it is called benign; the tremor is not accompanied by akinesia (slowness of movement), rigidity or gait disturbance, as occurs in Parkinson's disease (see Chapter 5), and so does not cause major disability.

Benign essential tremor often runs in families. A strange characteristic feature of the condition is that it may be helped dramatically but temporarily by the ingestion of alcohol.

Benign essential tremor cannot be 'cured', but can be eased considerably by drugs taken on a day-to-day basis. Treatment is, however, quite different from that of Parkinson's disease. Some of the drugs used are propranolol, phenobarbitone and primidone.

Infections

Encephalitis lethargica is a viral infection of the brain which occurred in epidemics from around 1915 to 1925. Although patients often seemed to recover from the acute infection many sufferers developed Parkinsonism over the next few years. The Parkinsonism differed from that of idiopathic Parkinson's disease in several respects: greasiness of the skin over the face, marked salivation, more prevalent dementia and oculogyric crises. Oculogyric crises are attacks of involuntary movement of both eyes, usually upwards, and sometimes accompanied by similar movement of the head. The attacks last for seconds to many minutes or even hours.

Parkinsonism developed after *encephalitis lethargica* because the virus produced damage to the part of the brain that is also affected in idiopathic Parkinson's disease. However, *encephalitis lethargica* has now virtually died out, so new cases of post-encephalitic Parkinsonism hardly, if ever, occur. We have no evidence that idiopathic Parkinson's disease is caused by a virus (see Chapter 4).

Drug-induced Parkinsonism

Certain drugs produce chemical changes in the brain that are very similar to those of Parkinson's disease. Consequently, treatment with these drugs, particularly in the long term and at high dosage, may produce features very similar to those of Parkinson's disease. Some of these drugs, which are often used in psychiatry, are listed in the accompanying box and should be avoided, as far as possible, by someone with idiopathic Parkinson's disease because they are likely to make the symptoms worse.

Someone with drug-induced Parkinsonism will usually improve if treatment with the responsible drug is ceased. Sometimes, however, the Parkinsonian features persist despite cessation of treatment. In addition, these drugs can produce other sorts of movement disorder that are quite different from Parkinson's disease and that are more likely to persist when the treatment is withdrawn. The commonest of these is called tardive dyskinesia.

Patients with drug-induced Parkinsonism who need to continue treatment with the responsible drug can benefit from anti-Parkinsonian drugs, in the same way as do patients with idiopathic Parkinson's disease.

Drugs that may cause Parkinsonism

- reserpine
- haloperidol
- tetrabenazine
- chlorpromazine
- fluphenazine
- prochlorperazine
- flupenthixol

Poisonous substances

Rarely, poisoning by substances such as carbon monoxide or manganese may produce a Parkinsonian condition.

Degenerative diseases of the nervous system

The shaking and difficulty in movement seen in idiopathic Parkinson's disease are due to abnormalities in certain regions of the brain, known as the basal ganglia, that are involved in the control of movement. In Parkinson's disease the major abnormality occurs because of loss of cells that produce dopamine. The abnormalities of the basal ganglia in Parkinson's disease are discussed further in Chapter 3.

Damage to the basal ganglia may also occur in other diseases that are not true Parkinson's disease, although in these conditions the cell death is not particularly restricted to cells that produce dopamine. The features of these diseases may very much mimic those of Parkinson's disease because the same brain regions are affected; however, because the damage is not confined to the cells that produce dopamine, these conditions do not respond so well to treatment with dopamine replacement as does idiopathic Parkinson's disease (see Chapter 8). Some of these diseases also damage brain regions outside the basal ganglia, so that the affected patients show special features in addition to those of Parkinsonism. For example, progressive supranuclear palsy is one condition in which the signs of Parkinson's disease in the arms and legs are accompanied by paralysis of eye movements so that the patients have particular difficulty in looking upwards or downwards. The Shy-Drager syndrome combines features of Parkinsonism with damage to a particular part of the nervous system, known as the autonomic nervous system. Because the autonomic nervous system is involved in maintaining blood pressure on changing from a sitting to a standing position, patients with Shy-Drager syndrome tend to have severe dizziness on standing because the blood pressure drops; they also show problems in control of the bladder and sexual impotence. Occasionally, some of these autonomic symptoms, such as fall in blood pressure on standing, may occur in uncomplicated idiopathic Parkinson's disease; treatment with levodopa and dopamine agonists tends to make these symptoms worse (see Chapter 8).

These Parkinsonian degenerative conditions have a variety of names, depending on the precise brain region that is affected by damage; they include corticostriatonigral degeneration, progressive supranuclear palsy, multiple system atrophy, Shy-Drager syndrome and olivopontocerebellar degeneration. Unlike Parkinson's disease, some of these conditions are passed on in families.

Stroke

One cause of stroke is a blockage (a thrombosis, or blood clot) in a main blood vessel (artery) to the brain, leading to permanent and irreversible damage (an infarction) to the area of the brain supplied by that blood vessel. With advancing age the risk of stroke increases because thickening of the artery walls causes the insides of the vessels to narrow, this process being called arteriosclerosis or hardening of the arteries; it is particularly common in people with high blood pressure or people who smoke cigarettes.

In a stroke the onset is usually sudden and obvious. However sometimes the vessel narrowing can occur slowly over several years, so that the circulation of blood to the brain diminishes gradually. This causes the brain damage to occur slowly and progressively. When this occurs patients can develop signs similar to those of true Parkinson's disease; the term arteriosclerotic Parkinsonism is therefore sometimes used for this condition. Patients with arteriosclerotic Parkinsonism often stand and walk in a similar fashion to people with Parkinson's disease, but tremor is usually absent and dementia is more common. Moreover, doctors can often detect signs of damage in other parts of the brain when they examine their patients. The condition does not usually respond to dopamine replacement.

Head trauma

A single severe head injury, such as follows a road traffic accident, can produce permanent brain damage. Such patients may develop abnormalities of gait and posture that superficially resemble Parkinson's disease. However there are usually signs of more diffuse damage to the brain, including major abnormalities of memory and general intellectual ability. Repeated minor trauma to the head, such as occurs in professional boxers, may produce a more gradual onset of diffuse brain damage that more closely resembles idiopathic Parkinson's disease (punch-drunkenness). However, tremor is usually inconspicuous, whereas intellectual decline is more common. The condition does not respond to dopamine replacement because the damage is more widespread than simply to the cells containing dopamine.

Normal pressure hydrocephalus

Cerebrospinal fluid is a clear liquid that bathes the brain. It is continually produced and reabsorbed in the brain so that a slow circulation occurs, similar to the circulation of the blood. Sometimes, conditions occur that interfere with this circulation so that there is a build-up of fluid and pressure inside the head.

One such condition is called normal pressure hydrocephalus, and it occurs particularly in the elderly. The features of this condition include disturbance of gait, dementia and incontinence. Because the condition occurs in the elderly, and often shows as disturbance of gait, it may be mistaken for idiopathic Parkinson's disease. Doctors are, however, alerted by the three main features of this condition described above. It can be diagnosed by a brain scan and is treated by a small neurosurgical operation.

Arthritis

When Parkinson's disease develops slowly and gradually, and tremor is not a prominent symptom, patients may complain of generalized slowness, stiffness, aching and difficulty in getting about. It is easy to misdiagnose these complaints as generalized arthritis or rheumatism. This is particularly so because both conditions are common in the elderly and both may produce a change in posture and ability to walk. Not all patients with Parkinson's disease have tremor, especially in the early stages, so the diagnosis may be delayed until a tremor develops or someone thinks of the diagnosis.

Thyroid disease and other metabolic disorders

Underactivity of the thyroid gland produces general slowing of all bodily activities, including movement. Although the resemblance is only superficial, this slowing up of movement may be mistaken for Parkinson's disease, or vice versa. An underactive thyroid is, however, important to recognize because it can be easily treated by taking regular thyroid tablets. Sometimes the body can develop changes in other important chemicals, such as the blood level of calcium, or copper (Wilson's disease), which can cause problems similar to those of Parkinson's disease. These conditions are easily diagnosed by a simple blood test.

Other causes of tremor

Some of the more common causes of tremor, such as benign essential tremor, have been discussed above. Other neurological diseases may also produce tremor, but the features of these tremors are usually quite distinct from those of Parkinsonism. Thus, for example, multiple sclerosis may produce damage to the cerebellum within the brain, which leads to tremor. However, unlike most cases of Parkinsonian tremor, the tremor of cerebellar disease is much worse when the hands are used than when they are rested. Huntington's disease is an inherited condition that is accompanied by involuntary movements of the whole body. Again, these movements, which are known as chorea, are quite different from those seen in uncomplicated Parkinson's disease.

It must be stressed that neither multiple sclerosis nor Huntington's disease has any relationship to Parkinson's disease, and can usually be distinguished easily by the examining doctor. Interestingly, however, the movements of chorea (but not the disease of Huntington's disease) can be produced by large doses of levodopa and become more pronounced in those patients who have had Parkinson's disease for a number of years.

2

Who gets Parkinson's disease?

When you are told you have Parkinson's disease you may ask 'What have I done to get this?' The short answer is nothing. A second common question is 'Is there something special about me?' and again, the simple answer is no. You may then ask 'Well, in that case, what causes it?' The answer to this, which is discussed further in Chapter 4, appears to be something in the environment but nothing that you could necessarily avoid. At the present time, a lot of research is being carried out to determine the cause of the disease and the reason or reasons why some people are particularly susceptible. Advances are constantly being made, but you should remember, when you read this chapter and Chapter 4, that we do not have the exact answers to these questions at the moment.

How common is Parkinson's disease?

Parkinson's disease is very common and has probably been around for a long time, certainly before James Parkinson described it in 1817. It has been reported from most countries of the world, although most research has been carried out in Europe and the United States, so most of the available information concerns people in those countries. It does appear to be less common in China and Japan than in the white races of the West, but the exact reason for this is unknown. It has been suggested (but not proven) that Parkinson's disease is caused by some toxic substance in the environment, produced by industry. The lower incidence in China, which is much more of a farming community, could then be due to less of this toxic substance in the environment. At the moment, however, this is little more than an inspired guess. Some people believe that Parkinson's disease is rare in the black races of the United States and Africa, but the evidence for this is not very convincing.

Incidence of Parkinson's disease in selected countries

Area	Prevalence/ 100,000	Study/Year
Leeds, England	60	Garland, 1952
Boston, USA	65	Schwab & England, 1958
Goteberg, Sweden	70	Broman, 1964
Carlisle, England	114.5	Brewis et al., 1961
Wellington, New Zealand	106	Pollock & Hornsbrook, 1962
Iceland	169.5	Godmundsson, 1963
Rochester, USA	157	Nobrega et al., 1965
Gippsland, Australia	85	Jenkins, 1965
Turku, Finland	120.1	Martilla & Rinne, 1971
Sardinia	65.6	Rosati et al., 1972

Parkinson's disease affects approximately one in every 500 people. This means that, at any one time, there are approximately 100,000 people with Parkinson's disease in the United Kingdom and over 300,000 in the United States. Parkinson's disease is more common than multiple sclerosis, although not as common as epilepsy.

Most people develop Parkinson's disease between the ages of 50 and 80 years. There is no doubt that it does affect younger people in their 30s and 40s, and even children although it is rare under the age of about 30 years. However, it becomes more common as people get older, so that it affects about one person in 60 between the ages of 70 and 80 years. Interestingly, it may become less common again after the age of 80.

These figures tell us how many people in the country have the disease at any one time, regardless of how long they have had it. But another way of telling the frequency of a disease is to count the number of people who develop the condition for the first time each year. For Parkinson's disease, the calculation shows that about 9,000 people develop the disease each year in the United Kingdom. Taken through a whole lifetime, everybody has a one in 40 chance of developing Parkinson's disease at some time.

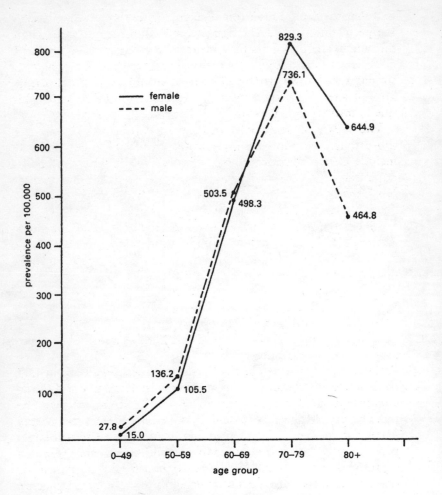

Prevalence of Parkinson's disease by age and sex (Finland, 1971)

Does it shorten life?

Parkinson's disease is not a fatal disease like the more serious forms of cancer. However, if you examine the death rates among people who suffer from any chronic disease, including diabetes, high blood pressure, bronchitis and arthritis, you will find that the death rate is, on average, higher than in people who are perfectly healthy. The figures for Parkinson's disease are in the same category. This may mean that a Parkinsonian patient has a risk of death two or three times higher than someone of a similar age. However, you must bear in mind that most people around age 60 would expect to live for many more years and this is also true of patients with Parkinson's disease.

The causes of death in patients with Parkinson's disease are those that are found in any chronically disabled person, and include chest infections and general weakness. The drug levodopa has considerably reduced the long-term disability and so has increased the life expectancy, such that the average age at death in patients with Parkinson's disease is 70–75 years; however there is a very wide range, and the figures are not much different from the average population who do not have Parkinson's disease. The majority of people with Parkinson's disease die of some completely unrelated condition.

Does it affect particular sorts of people?

Parkinson's disease is equally common in men and women. It does not seem to occur in clusters in any particular parts of the country, so no area seems any more at risk than any other. The risk of contracting the disease does not seem to be related to any particular job or social status. Certain drugs and poisons can produce a condition very much like Parkinson's disease (see also Chapters 1 and 4); however, the risk of contracting idiopathic or true Parkinson's disease is not affected by any previous exposure to normal medication nor to X-rays, power stations, particular sorts of animals or alcohol intake. As discussed further in Chapter 4, you are no more likely to get Parkinson's disease because you have pursued a particular lifestyle; in particular, you will not acquire Parkinson's disease because you have been subject to stress, physical exhaustion or overwork.

But although there is nothing you can do to avoid the onset of Parkinson's disease, there do seem to be some interesting features to suggest that particular sorts of people may be at risk. This information has been acquired by questioning people with Parkinson's disease about their characteristics before they developed the disease. These sorts of studies have shown that people with Parkinson's disease smoke on average less through their life than do non-Parkinsonians; in particular, there are many more people with Parkinson's disease who have never smoked at any time in their life than can be found in the general population. One explanation for this is that something in cigarette smoke protects the brain from the damage that causes Parkinson's disease. However, you would be well advised not to start smoking in order to protect yourself against Parkinson's disease or to delay its progression. There are very many other conditions in medicine that are caused or worsened by smoking and these far outweigh the benefit that smoking may give to Parkinson's disease. Moreover, the observation that Parkinson's disease is more common in non-smokers does not necessarily mean that smoking protects you against Parkinson's disease. The association between Parkinson's disease and non-smoking may occur because of the personality type of the person who later gets Parkinson's disease. The Parkinsonian patient has been described as more introverted, rather mentally inflexible and prone to depression. These personality features seem to be present prior to the onset of Parkinson's disease, so they are not caused by it; rather, they seem to indicate that particular personality types are prone to Parkinson's disease and this personality type tends not to smoke.

Some people believe that the personality type exists in Parkinson's disease because the brain changes began very many years earlier, but others think that it simply shows the susceptibility of certain sorts of people. This intriguing question is unanswered at the present time, but is discussed further in Chapter 4.

How quickly does the disease progress?

Parkinson's disease does have a tendency to get worse, but at a very variable rate. Maybe one in ten of all patients show little progression of the condition and appear to be perfectly controlled, even after many years. For the rest, existing symptoms tend to progress and new symptoms of Parkinson's disease develop. However, this progression is over the course of years rather than over the course of months. The condition does not suddenly worsen; there are no 'overnight surprises'.

For those who do get worse, symptoms which at first affect only one hand may begin to affect both; walking may become affected; akinesia (slowness of movement), rigidity or tremor may become prominent when previously it was not; and some of the other symptoms, described in Chapters 6 and 7, may develop for the first time. You should realize, though, that most of these symptoms can be kept under control by adjustment of treatment so that, for most people, persistent problems do not develop for many years, provided they see their doctor at regular intervals. When greater problems do develop, they usually do so after seven to ten years of the disease, and consist of response fluctuations (Chapter 8) and memory difficulties (Chapter 6).

In some ways, the outlook is rather better for the younger patient than for the older. For the younger group, the various treatments appear to be more effective; difficulty in walking, due to problems with posture and gait, are less troublesome in these patients and the development of dementia is rarer. However, younger people are more prone to the development of response fluctuations and dyskinesias. For people of any age, those who develop tremor early may have a better outlook than those who begin with prominent akinesia or rigidity. Such people may have no symptoms other than tremor for several years.

3

What's gone wrong?

Parkinson's disease is mainly a problem of movement, but it is not a disease of the muscles. To make a movement, we obviously need the muscles in order to move the arms and legs; however, when we decide to move, the signal originates in the brain and reaches the muscles through a network of nerves that act like telephone wires, transmitting the message from one part of the body (the brain) to another (the muscles).

Occasionally, a movement occurs through the contraction of a single muscle; more often, however, many muscles are involved. Even a simple movement, such as lifting up one arm, requires the contraction of several muscles, including, in this example, those at the shoulder, the elbow and the forearm. To make the movement properly, each muscle has to be contracted to just the right degree, not too much and not too little. Thus, separate signals have to be passed down to each muscle at the same time, indicating precisely the extent and timing of that particular contraction. The situation is even more complicated when we wish to make a movement that involves different parts of the body. For example, in walking, we not only have to co-ordinate the muscular contractions within one leg, but also have to co-ordinate the movements of the two legs together. Furthermore we have to vary the messages across time. For example, we may need to vary the speed of walking; we will need to alter direction slightly, depending on obstacles that cross our path; and we may wish to start, stop, slow down and speed up.

Dopamine and the brain

The co-ordination of the nerve messages to muscles in different parts of the body occurs within the brain. One particular part of the brain that is important for this co-ordination is called the

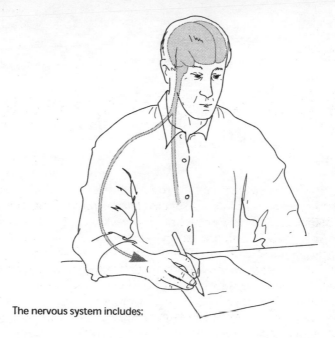

The nervous system includes:

Central nervous system:
• Brain
• Spinal cord

Peripheral nervous system:
• Nerves carry messages
  between central nervous
  system and organs and tissues
  such as muscle (see detail below)

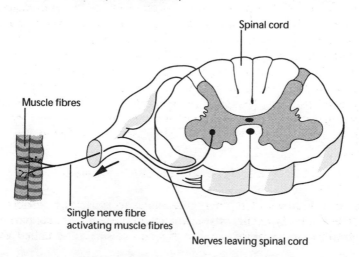

Spinal cord

Muscle fibres

Single nerve fibre
activating muscle fibres

Nerves leaving spinal cord

How the nervous system controls movement

basal ganglia, and it sits more or less in the centre of the brain, at the top of the 'stalk' of the 'mushroom' you can see in the diagram on page 17.

When we decide to make a movement the thinking part of the brain (the managing director) sends its instructions to the basal ganglia (the executive), and the basal ganglia then co-ordinate a series of messages that pass out, at the right time, to each part of the nervous system (the telephone network). The correct timing of the arrival of these messages at the individual muscles (the workforce) causes the muscles to contract in the right order and with the right force; using another metaphor, this is similar to the activities of the members of a symphony orchestra, in which each member contributes to the whole symphony.

Although we tend to speak of the basal ganglia as a single unit, the term in fact refers to several different units, which themselves act together. Not only are the basal ganglia involved in co-ordinating activities between the thinking parts of the brain and the nerves to the muscles but they also send messages to and from each other in order to carry out their necessary activities. The brain and nervous system consist of a series of cells, rather like individual wires; messages are sent from one cell to another cell, in a similar way to the transfer of messages to a computer across wires. Now, while there are certainly some similarities between a brain and a computer, there are many differences, and one important difference for our purposes is the fact that messages are transmitted through the brain using chemicals that are made within the nerve cells. The nerve cell requires these chemicals in order to transmit messages to another cell, and without them messages will not be transmitted effectively from one nerve cell to the next.

The brain uses a variety of different chemicals to transmit messages across nerves – dopamine is one, acetylcholine and noradrenaline are two others. In the basal ganglia one of the most important chemicals for the transmission of messages is dopamine, and therein lies the basic fault of Parkinson's disease. Within the basal ganglia, the cells that produce dopamine work less well and eventually die off, and the remaining cells then cannot generate a strong enough message for it to pass from one cell to the next, the result being that the basal ganglia cannot work effectively. As a consequence, the system that co-ordinates movement through the body breaks down, and this leads directly to the symptoms of Parkinson's disease. The main area affected is called the substantia nigra because, when stained in a particular way and examined under the microscope, it shows up as a blackened area (nigra meaning black) against the rest of the brain, which is light grey.

What effect does lack of dopamine have?

The loss of dopamine from the basal ganglia means that the messages transmitted from the thinking part of the brain cannot be translated into a form that can be passed out to the individual muscles. This means that you may well know what you intend to do, but the muscles fail to respond to your intentions. It is not the case, however, that no messages get through at all; the problem is one of co-ordinating all the messages together. This means that sometimes you may be able to move your arms or legs quite normally, but on other occasions the message simply does not get through. The lack of dopamine does not usually produce any weakness of the muscles themselves. Although many patients do feel weak, this sensation usually results from an inability to get their act together; that is, they are unable to get a message to the muscle to tell it to pull hard enough. This inability to get messages through to the muscles is the major problem underlying what is called akinesia (slowness in starting movement).

But if the difficulty is in transmitting messages, why are there problems such as rigidity and tremor when the limbs are not being used? Surely the co-ordination of messages is not necessary when the limbs are completely at rest? This is a false assumption, though. The basal ganglia are continually in action, even when the limbs are resting, ensuring that the right messages get through and that false messages do not. The origin of rigidity and tremor is rather complicated, but can be thought of as a problem in blocking false messages. Just as the basal ganglia cannot let the right messages through in Parkinson's disease, they also fail to block the wrong messages; this means that the muscles are working, either becoming stiffer or contracting rhythmically, when they should not be.

What is wrong with the dopamine cells?

The nerve cells in the substantia nigra, and sometimes elsewhere

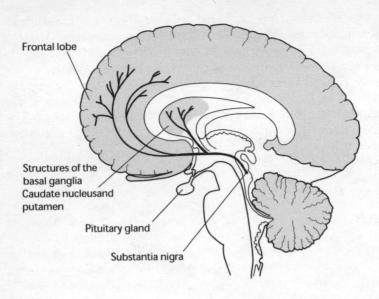

Frontal lobe

Structures of the
basal ganglia
Caudate nucleusand
putamen

Pituitary gland

Substantia nigra

Section of mid-brain

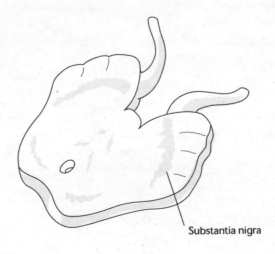

Substantia nigra

Location of the basal ganglia and substantia nigra in the brain

in the brain, become damaged because there is a build-up of protein substance within the cells, and this ultimately destroys them. When these cells are examined under the microscope, the damage shows up as a very typical appearance known as the Lewy body, named after Lewy who first described the appearance in the Parkinsonian brain in 1912. Lewy bodies look like round darkened circles, with a light halo around them. The Lewy body is important to doctors and researchers because, when it is present in large numbers, it provides definite evidence that the brain is damaged by Parkinson's disease.

Is the rest of the brain affected?

There is no doubt that the major problems lie within the dopamine cells of the basal ganglia, which are responsible for the problems in movement so characteristic of Parkinson's disease. However there are also less prominent changes in other parts of the brain, although researchers are not sure of the clinical effect of damage in these areas.

The basal ganglia are the main site of dopamine cells. Other parts of the brain contain cells with different chemicals, acetylcholine or noradrenaline, and these are also partially damaged in Parkinson's disease. In addition, the kind of damage that occurs in the basal ganglia is sometimes seen to a lesser degree in other parts of the brain, including the thinking parts in the cap of the 'mushroom' you can see in the diagram on page 20.

The loss of dopamine is the major cause of the problems of movement, which is why dopamine replacement helps so much and is the mainstay of treatment (see Chapter 8). But damage to other chemical systems or other parts of the brain may be responsible for some of the other features of Parkinson's disease, including problems with memory, depression, control of urine and control of blood pressure. Damage to these other areas is currently under research.

How is Parkinson's disease diagnosed?

Damage to the dopamine-containing cells by Lewy bodies can only be detected by examining the brain under a microscope, and so can only be done after a person has died. But it is now possible to detect loss of dopamine from the basal ganglia during life, using techniques known as positron emission tomography (PET) and single photon emission tomography (SPET). These work like a very elaborate brain scanner. However, the necessary machinery is available in only relatively few cities around the world and is used largely for research purposes. It may be that in the future PET and SPET scanning or something similar will become more widely available so that it can be used to make a diagnosis of Parkinson's disease in an ordinary hospital or clinic, but at present this cannot be accommodated. As there is no other way of visualizing the damage to the dopamine cells or of picking up the loss of the chemical dopamine from the basal ganglia, this means that the diagnosis of Parkinson's disease has to be made clinically; that is, by your doctor taking a detailed history of your symptoms and by performing an examination that picks up the tell-tale signs of Parkinson's disease and detects no signs that indicate an alternative diagnosis.

Why, then, do you sometimes have to undergo special tests? The reason for this is because your doctor wants to rule out other diseases. Although we cannot pick up positive evidence of Parkinson's disease from X-rays, blood tests or any other investigation, some other conditions, which may be confused with Parkinson's disease, do show up in these tests. Your doctor may therefore ask for such tests because he is uncertain about the diagnosis and wants to be sure that there is no evidence of an alternative diagnosis. (The sort of conditions that can sometimes be confused with Parkinson's disease are discussed in Chapter 1.)

Your doctor will rule out some of these conditions, such as benign essential tremor, from your history and his examination. He will elicit your history of previous encephalitis, if there is one, and will ask you for details of your medication to see if any of these could be producing signs similar to those of Parkinson's disease. His examination will often show signs that indicate the diagnosis to be one of the degenerative diseases, distinct from Parkinson's disease, and his ability to make this diagnosis may be helped by asking for details of similar diseases in your relatives. He will want to know if you have had any serious head trauma and whether you have ever been a professional boxer.

He may undertake a series of blood tests to rule out problems with thyroid disease, Wilson's disease and other problems with blood chemistry. He may then ask you to have two special investigations, a CT (or MRI) scan and an EEG. These two tests can provide positive evidence of previous stroke, Alzheimer's disease or normal pressure hydrocephalus.

But if you are not asked to undergo any of these tests you should not be alarmed. Often the diagnosis of Parkinson's disease is obvious to the doctor when he first examines you, and there can be no confusion with any other diagnosis. The tests are thus only used when there seems to be a need to rule out other conditions.

CT and MRI scans

For a computerized tomography or CT scan you are asked to lie flat on your back on a couch, and are then wheeled towards the CT scanning machine so that the top part of the head is contained within the opening of the scanner. You are then simply required to stay as still as possible during the scanning procedure, which takes 10–20 minutes. You will experience no pain during the procedure, and the only awareness of the scan will be a clicking or whirring sound. Some patients who are particularly prone to claustrophobia may feel a little anxious, but this is seldom a troublesome problem. You may be given an injection into your arm of a kind of X-ray dye, in order to produce clearer pictures; this discomfort is no worse than that of having blood taken. No other pain is involved in the procedure.

Magnetic resonance imaging is another sort of brain scan. It is similar to CT scans but works by magnetism rather than X-rays. However, from your point of view, the procedure is very similar to that of CT scanning except that you should not have anything magnetic on your person and you may be asked not to have the scan if you have metal inside your body from, for example, shrapnel, some sorts of surgical operations and heart pacemakers. MRI scanning is more recent than CT scanning but is now fairly freely available. You may be asked to have either kind of scan.

EEG

The electroencephalograph or EEG is a method of picking up

the electrical activity of the brain. Several leads are placed on the scalp, often utilizing a device similar to a hairnet. The leads are then attached to a sensitive machine that is capable of picking up the brainwaves through the scalp and bones of the skull. No electric shocks are given, and the procedure is totally painless. Sometimes you are asked to take deep breaths, or you might be asked to watch a flashing light, but there is generally no discomfort.

This test is sometimes used to pick up evidence of degenerative diseases distinct from Parkinson's disease, such as Alzheimer's disease.

4

What causes Parkinson's disease?

We know that the symptoms of Parkinson's disease are mostly due to loss of dopamine from the basal ganglia, as described in Chapter 3. However, this is not a cause; to establish a cause we would need to know what caused the loss of dopamine in the first place, and the answer to this question is unknown. In this chapter, however, we will discuss some of the main theories that have been developed from continuing research. The quantity of research being carried out into Parkinson's disease at the present time is probably greater than at any time in the past, and there is a prospect of finding the cause, a permanent cure, or both. At the time of writing, however, that cause must remain only a theory.

If you have Parkinson's disease, this chapter will not help you a great deal in your day-to-day life, but it will answer many questions that may have sprung to your mind. In addition, it will hopefully allay some of your anxieties about things in your own life that you had thought may have been important in causing Parkinson's disease.

Is Parkinson's disease caused by a virus?

We know that virus infections of the brain can produce a condition very similar to Parkinson's disease, this condition being known as post-encephalitic Parkinsonism (see Chapter 1). The features of post-encephalitic Parkinsonism are different in many respects from idiopathic Parkinson's disease, but the finding that a virus infection can produce symptoms similar to Parkinson's disease has prompted the idea that idiopathic Parkinson's disease may also be caused by a virus. Unfortunately no such virus has been found. In addition, despite the evidence from post-encephalitic Parkinsonism, there is also some reason to believe that idiopathic Parkinson's disease is not caused by a virus.

- Firstly, we continue to see new cases of Parkinson's disease, even though *encephalitis lethargica* now seems to have died out. No other brain infection apart from *encephalitis lethargica* has ever been shown to produce a condition like Parkinson's disease, so we have no reason to suspect any other virus.

- The Parkinsonism that results from *encephalitis lethargica* is different in many respects from that of idiopathic Parkinson's disease, so the two conditions are not really comparable.

- The changes that take place in the brain in post-encephalitic Parkinsonism are distinctly different from those of idiopathic Parkinson's disease, even though both conditions have loss of dopamine from the basal ganglia.

- When we look at the changes in the brain in Parkinson's disease, we do not see any of the changes that we know occur with ordinary virus infections.

- Finally, no one has ever succeeded in giving Parkinson's disease to laboratory animals by injection of substances derived from patients with Parkinson's disease, even though this sort of disease spread has been successful for other brain diseases thought to be caused by viruses.

At present, therefore, we can only conclude that there is no evidence whatever that a virus is responsible for idiopathic Parkinson's disease, even though brain infection can produce a condition that looks very similar.

Is Parkinson's disease inherited?

Most people, when told that they have Parkinson's disease, are anxious to know whether they will pass on the condition to their children. Indeed, people are often able to identify someone else in the family who has suffered from it. Sometimes, though, it turns out that these family relatives did not have Parkinson's disease but benign essential tremor, which is easily confused with Parkinson's disease and which is passed on in families (see Chapter 1). In other cases, however, it does appear that there is a family relative with true Parkinson's disease.

This latter type of family history is obtained from approximately one in ten patients with Parkinson's disease. Put another way, the risk of Parkinson's disease developing within the immediate family is approximately double that of the general population. Clearly, this raises the question that the condition is inherited. In a few rare families, with many relatives affected by Parkinson's disease, a faulty gene has been found to be responsible. In these families, the condition is inherited. However, the faulty gene has not been found in the vast majority of people with Parkinson's. Moreover, studies have examined a large numbers of pairs of twins (who have identical genetic inheritance) and found that the twin was no more likely to develop Parkinson's disease than if he were a member of a different family. This argues against the theory that the disease is inherited in any simple way in the majority of cases.

But it is possible to inherit a predisposition to a disease, if not the disease itself, and this may be true of Parkinson's disease. In other words, your genetic background may render you more susceptible to something in the environment which itself produces the disease. Recent research suggests that this sort of susceptibility may be inherited in Parkinson's disease. In general, though, you can be content that you will not pass on the disease in any predictable way to any of your descendants. If they do develop the disease, it is mostly because it is common in the general population anyway, and perhaps because they are rather more susceptible.

So why is the condition more common in families of Parkinsonian patients? The answer is most likely that the condition is caused by something in the environment and that people from the same family tend to share the same environment. You can conclude from this that there is no major risk that you will pass on the disease to your family and, if their tendency to develop the disease is increased, it is mostly because they breathe the same air and eat the same food as you do.

Is Parkinson's disease caused by pollution?

We have discussed the finding that Parkinson's disease may run in families but that usually it seems not, in itself, to be inherited, and that the explanation of this discrepancy may lie in something in the environment that causes Parkinson's disease, combined with a predisposition to its effects. As a result of these observations, many researchers have been interested in the possibility that the damage occurs through poisoning of the dopamine cells of the basal ganglia from a toxic substance in the environment. This possibility has been increased markedly with the discovery that the Parkinsonian condition can be produced by a toxin known as MPTP.

In the late 1970s drug addicts in California were making their own drugs as a cheap alternative to heroin. One of these addicts, a 23-year-old student, started to become ill; over several days he developed tremor, rigidity and akinesia, so that eventually he presented an appearance that was indistinguishable from Parkinson's disease, even to doctors. He was treated with anti-Parkinsonian drugs, and improved dramatically. Some time later, though, he died from an overdose of other drugs. When his brain was examined at post-mortem, there was found to be severe damage to the dopamine-containing cells in the basal ganglia, similar to that seen in Parkinson's disease. He was obviously very young to be developing idiopathic Parkinson's disease, so the doctors suspected that his condition was caused by the drugs that he was taking. They analysed the material that he had been making, and found that it contained a by-product known as MPTP. And further research showed that MPTP was capable of producing severe damage to the dopamine-containing cells in the basal ganglia.

Following that first case, many other drug addicts have developed a similar Parkinsonian syndrome after injecting themselves with drugs contaminated by MPTP. All of these people developed symptoms and signs that could not be distinguished from idiopathic Parkinson's disease, and they all responded to anti-Parkinsonian drugs. In addition, some of the people developed the response fluctuations, including on-off swings, that occur in idiopathic Parkinson's disease. Furthermore, one person who developed the MPTP Parkinsonian syndrome was not a drug addict; instead he was a chemist who had acquired the condition from working with MPTP at a drug firm – presumably he had become poisoned by breathing the substance or from contamination of the skin.

You should not jump to the conclusion from these facts that idiopathic Parkinson's disease is caused by MPTP poisoning. Firstly, MPTP does not seem to be around in the environment; it was produced in California only as an artificial substance during the making of an illicit drug. Secondly, the changes that occur in the brain are a little different from those of idiopathic Parkinson's disease, even though there is severe damage to the dopamine-containing cells. Of course, we do not know whether the changes in the brain would be identical if the MPTP poisoning occurred gradually over a much longer period of time, or if it occurred in people of an older age group. Nevertheless, these possibilities are very unlikely; therefore we do not believe that MPTP causes idiopathic Parkinson's disease.

These patients have shown us, however, that poisonous substances can produce illnesses very similar to Parkinson's disease, and have thus caused many researchers to ask if the disease can be caused by any other poison present in the environment and not yet identified. Some studies have suggested that people with Parkinson's have had a greater exposure throughout life to certain chemical substances, such as weed-killers, insecticides, chemical solvents and well-water. A great deal of research is being carried out at present in order to answer this question more definitely.

Is Parkinson's disease due to getting older?

Parkinson's disease is commoner in older people, but that does not prove that it is caused just by aging. Indeed, it seems to become rather less common after the age of 80, and we would not expect this if the disease were simply due to getting old.

To some degree, though, aging probably does increase your risk, even though some other factor has to occur for you to get the disease. As we get older, the brain tends to show changes similar to those of Parkinson's disease, but in a much milder form. For example, Lewy bodies tend to occur, affecting up to one in ten people over the age of 60; however, the changes are milder than those that occur in Parkinson's disease. Furthermore, the levels of dopamine in the basal ganglia get gradually less as we get older. In order to show signs of Parkinson's disease you need to lose more than 60–80 per cent of the dopamine from your basal ganglia, so there is quite a considerable reserve capacity; when the levels fall with increasing age, however, there is less reserve, so Parkinson's disease may develop more readily when something in the environment damages the remaining dopamine cells.

Other people have suggested that the effect of age works in a different way. They have suggested that the poisoning occurs earlier in life, but it does not show because it does not reduce the dopamine levels by the 60–80 per cent necessary to show Parkinson's disease; however, the levels are lower than they otherwise would be. As the years go by, the levels drop even further as a result of natural aging so that, by about 60 years, they fall below the critical level and Parkinson's disease develops. If you did not experience such poisoning earlier in life, then you would show higher levels over the years and you might therefore get through life without a fall in dopamine sufficient for you to show the disease. This idea has been used to explain why people with Parkinson's disease seem to show certain personality characteristics for many years before they develop the disease; the idea is that the levels of dopamine are reduced enough to produce a change in personality but not to produce problems with movement. You should realize that this is an intriguing idea, but, regrettably, completely unproven. However, the research continues.

Some other changes can also occur with age. Older people are at greater risk of the development of Alzheimer's disease, a cause of severe memory loss. Just as we can find changes of Parkinson's disease in the brains of elderly people who do not seem to have Parkinson's disease, we can also see mild changes, similar to those of Alzheimer's disease, in people who do not seem to have Alzheimer's disease. It is very important to realize, though, that Parkinson's disease and Alzheimer's disease are quite different diseases, and you are not at risk of one just because you have the other. The two diseases can occur together, but this is probably no more than a coincidence. The question of memory disturbance in Parkinson's disease is answered further in Chapter 6.

Are some people more prone to the disease?

If Parkinson's disease is caused by some poison in the environment, why is it that not everyone develops it? We know that Parkinson's disease is widespread throughout the world, so presumably the poison – if there is one – is also found throughout the world. If everyone is exposed to it, you might expect that most people would be poisoned by it. The fact that they are not suggests that some people are more susceptible to the disease than others. But this susceptibility is likely to be built into the individual; it is not something to do with your lifestyle that has lowered your resistance.

We have discussed earlier in this chapter that the disease is not usually inherited in the way that some diseases – like haemophilia, the bleeding disorder – seem to be. But it may be that something in your inherited make-up has made you more vulnerable to substances in the environment that produce Parkinson's disease. This would mean that you were in no danger if you were not exposed to this environmental factor; however, if you were, then you would be more likely to develop the disease if your inherited make-up puts you at greater risk.

We know that identical twins have identical inherited genetic make-up. What explanation can be put forward for the situation where one of a pair of identical twins has Parkinson's disease and the other doesn't? It may be that both of them have developed a susceptibility to the disease but only one of them has been exposed to the necessary factor in the environment – or to a strong enough dose of it – to produce the disease. Some research has supported this idea. The body is normally equipped with a set of defence mechanisms that will destroy poisonous substances if they enter the body. This is in fact the way that the body gets rid of drugs, once they have been used. Some studies have shown that these defence mechanisms may not be quite so efficient in Parkinson's disease as they usually are. This means that a toxic substance in the environment may not be destroyed so quickly in such people as it is in the rest of the population, so that the effect of the poison is greater. Assuming that the poison produces Parkinson's disease, these inefficient defence mechanisms would increase your risk of developing the disease.

But can an inherited inefficient defence mechanism cause the personality differences that we have mentioned earlier in this chapter? The answer has to be no. It is not that the inefficient defence mechanisms produce the personality changes; neither is it necessarily that the personality changes are caused by the environmental toxin. The idea is that people who inherit these inefficient defence systems also tend to inherit the type of personality that is introverted and prone to depression – one does not cause the other, but they both tend to be inherited together.

As with all research theories, these ideas should be taken very much as unproven. Science usually moves step by step rather than in great leaps and bounds. Each piece of evidence is fitted together, hopefully to produce the ultimate answer. This point has not yet been reached but research continues to advance along the path towards it.

Can I avoid Parkinson's disease?

No one can advise you on the kind of life to lead in order to avoid getting Parkinson's disease – except to avoid getting older. However, if you already have Parkinson's disease, it is human nature to search for something in your past life that may have been responsible for developing the disease. Some people even feel personal blame because of past guilt, or they may blame others for causing a crisis in their life, which they feel sure is responsible for their Parkinson's disease. All these emotions are understandable, and indeed part of human nature; nevertheless, the ideas are virtually always untrue.

We know of nothing in your lifestyle that will affect your risk of getting Parkinson's disease. It is not affected by stress, physical exhaustion, overwork, pregnancy, alcohol, sex or social class. The disease affects the rich and poor alike, fitness fanatics as well as followers of a debauched lifestyle. As far as we know, diet is unimportant (although it may be important once you have developed Parkinson's disease – see Chapter 9).

One particular question that is often asked is whether a head injury in the past could have been responsible for the development of Parkinson's disease. We do know that a severe head injury, as might occur in a car crash, can produce brain damage and superficial features of Parkinson's disease. However, the two are usually readily distinguishable. Repeated mild trauma to the head, such as occurs in professional boxers, can also produce a Parkinsonian condition; again, however, the condition is usually distinguishable from idiopathic Parkinson's disease, and the history of head trauma is typically very prominent, and frequent over many years. The boxer Mohammed Ali has a Parkinsonian syndrome which may be partially caused by repeated head trauma.

In other people, a history of head injury prior to the development of Parkinson's disease is probably totally irrelevant. Many people with Parkinson's disease do report a head injury in the past, but people with many other sorts of diseases also report a head injury in the past. Indeed, head injuries are very common in the general population, whether or not they suffer from a disease, but they tend not to be remembered because people have no cause to do so. It is only when some other event, such as Parkinson's disease, develops that we scan through our past life and remember these occasions. Although some researchers have reported an increased incidence of head injury in the life of patients with Parkinson's disease, compared with the general population, there is really little to suggest that a head injury is involved as the cause of idiopathic Parkinson's disease.

What can we conclude?

Lewy, who described the Lewy body now named after him (one of the typical changes in the Parkinsonian brain), said in 1940: 'When I had investigated my first two dozen cases of Parkinson's, I was convinced that I knew where the cause of tremor and rigidity was located. When I had examined pathologically the seventh dozen of Parkinson brains, I was completely confused because you seem to be able to prove just as well one theory as the contrary one.' Things are no longer as bleak as that, but the final answer still evades us. However, I think we can be hopeful that the cause will be found, if not to help everyone who already has the disease, then at least those who might develop it in the future and hopefully others too.

5

Problems of movement

It has been well known since the original descriptions of *paralysis agitans* by James Parkinson that Parkinson's disease affects particularly the ability to move. The difficulty in movement is caused not because of some muscle weakness (although patients may feel generally weak) but because of a difficulty in co-ordinating the action of different muscle groups. This inco-ordination is produced by abnormalities in the parts of the brain that co-ordinate movement. Doctors recognize three principal types of movement problem in Parkinson's disease:

- Akinesia
- Rigidity
- Tremor

In addition, a number of other types of difficulty in movement may occur as a result of drug treatment or in patients who have had the disease for many years.

Akinesia, rigidity and tremor may begin on one side of the body and, in some patients, remain limited to one side for a long time. In most patients, however, the condition progresses to involve both arms and both legs, although to varying degrees. As the condition develops it also affects posture and gait.

Akinesia and rigidity

Akinesia, or bradykinesia, means slowness of movement. Thus, although Parkinsonian sufferers may be able to carry out all tasks, it takes them considerably longer to do so and all the individual actions appear to take place at a much slower pace than would normally be the case. Of particular difficulty is the ability to start moving, even though the movement, once started, may also be carried out more slowly.

Sometimes different terms are used to describe these two different sorts of slowing down. Akinesia is often used to denote the difficulty in starting a movement, whilst bradykinesia is used to refer to the slowing of a movement once it has begun. For example, a patient may show akinesia in walking because he remains rooted to the spot, unable to take a step forward; however, he may also show bradykinesia of walking because his steps are smaller and he progresses at a slower rate. For practical purposes, both akinesia and bradykinesia cause similar problems so, in this book, the single term akinesia will be used to describe both sorts of problem.

The second major problem with movement is rigidity. Normally, the various muscles throughout the body are under slight contraction, even when they appear to be completely at rest. This slight contraction is known as muscle tone. If a person is asked to relax their limbs completely and another person moves the limb at one of the major joints, such as flexing the arm at the elbow, the resting muscle tone can be detected as a slight resistance to this movement. But when this manoeuvre is carried out on a patient with Parkinson's disease, the resistance is found to be much greater because of the presence of increased muscle tone, or muscular rigidity. The impression that is created when the limb is moved in this way has colourful terminology: 'lead pipe' rigidity refers to the general stiffness of the limb that changes little as the arm is moved. Often, however, one seems to encounter a series of 'catches' as the limb is moved, similar to the sensation of moving over a cog-wheel. Rigidity, particularly this 'cog-wheel' rigidity, is often felt in the arms of those with Parkinson's disease, but also affects the legs and neck.

The combination of akinesia and rigidity accounts for much of the disturbance of posture, gait and dexterity that affect the patient with Parkinson's disease. Apart from the involuntary tremor, which may or may not be present, many of the spontaneous movements of the body are lost.

Facial expression

The diminished movements of the face, particularly in response to social and emotional triggers, gives the impression of a

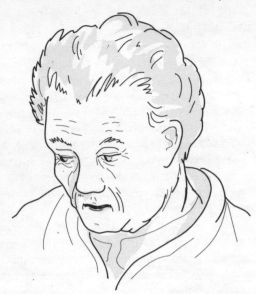

Mask-like or deadpan expression
and characteristic posture of the neck

Facial expression in Parkinson's disease

deadpan or mask-like face. In the early stages you may simply
see a reduced rate of spontaneous blinking or side-to-side eye
movements – these occur quite regularly in the normal individual. In more severe cases, though, there is loss of other
emotional expressions, including smiling and frowning. And in
the most advanced cases the face appears completely immobile.
The loss of movement, however, is not due to weakness, because
all muscles can be moved on command, albeit more slowly than
normal.

Speech

The ability to speak requires co-ordination not only of the
muscles in the larynx (voice box) but also the muscles that deal

with breathing and movement around the throat, tongue and nasal passages. To articulate words clearly, and to start and stop speaking without difficulty, requires an intricate co-ordination of all these different muscle groups. Since these muscles are also affected by akinesia in Parkinson's disease, it is not surprising that the condition is associated with abnormalities of speech.

In the milder cases there may be slight monotony, due to the lack of normal variation of pitch, together with a certain quietness and breathiness. In more severe cases the speech becomes slurred and difficult to understand. In the most severe cases speech may be unintelligible. These patients show great reduction in the volume and clarity of speech; their speech is often severely slurred and extremely quiet and monotonous. Their speech may also show a festinating (hurried) character, similar in principle to the difficulties in walking (see below), with the rapid repeated production of single unintelligible syllables. Fortunately, most patients with Parkinson's disease do not suffer from this severity of speech disturbance and are usually able to communicate effectively. For the minority with severe problems, however, the speech disturbance can interfere totally with effective oral communication.

Posture

The standing posture in Parkinson's disease is one of increased flexion (bending forwards) in the spine, arms and legs. This feature gives the characteristic stooped appearance, with the head and chest bent forward to a degree that depends on the severity of the illness. The arms are held partially bent at the elbows, with the hands poised towards the front. The knees are slightly bent. This posture tends to throw the centre of gravity forward so that the stability of the body is upset and patients easily fall over.

Similarly, while sitting, the Parkinsonian sufferer may appear slumped forward in the chair with the hands held close together on their lap, clearly unable to relax backwards in the chair. The forward tilt of the head on the neck may give the impression of constantly looking upwards at visitors, which, in fact, the Parkinsonian is obliged to do because of the altered posture caused by the disease.

Gait

Patients with Parkinson's disease experience particular difficulty in rising from a chair, especially a low one. Moreover, there is a tendency to fall over soon after standing because of difficulty in achieving balance rapidly enough after the initial sudden burst of movement required to gain the standing position.

Once standing, the akinesia causes considerable difficulty in starting to walk. People feel rooted to the spot or feel that their feet are stuck to the floor. Sometimes the first step can be made more easily by employing one of several kinds of tricks. Some people find benefit from marching on the spot and then taking a sudden step forward. Others find that they can take the first step if they begin counting in their head, and set themselves a target of taking their first step on reaching, for example, the number five. Others manage to move by telling themselves to throw the foot forward. All of these tricks seem to work by imparting a sudden burst of energy into the system to overcome the muscular resistance of that first step. A particularly ingenious method adopted by one patient involved attaching a dog lead to his shoe and passing the lead up his trouser leg, out of the top of the trousers and into his right hand. The first step was begun by pulling sharply on the lead with the right hand, which seemed to provide that extra impetus for the right foot to take its step.

The normal gait involves a fairly upright posture and a tendency for both arms to swing, particularly on brisk walking. On turning around, the head usually turns first, followed to a greater or lesser degree by spinning on one foot. The gait of the Parkinson's disease sufferer loses these features. In the early stages the only abnormality may be a failure to swing one arm on walking. But with a more advanced condition both arms fail to swing and are held semiflexed at the elbows, with the head thrown downwards and forwards as described above. Walking then tends to proceed by a series of small steps; the centre of gravity at chest level appears to be moving too fast for the movement of the feet, which always seem to be trying to catch up with the head and chest. If the feet catch, even on a small stretch of uneven ground, the person will readily fall forward.

Similar problems occur if they are required to stop suddenly or to change direction; patients with Parkinson's disease should be particularly careful under these circumstances as they are the times when falls most often occur. Turning is a particular

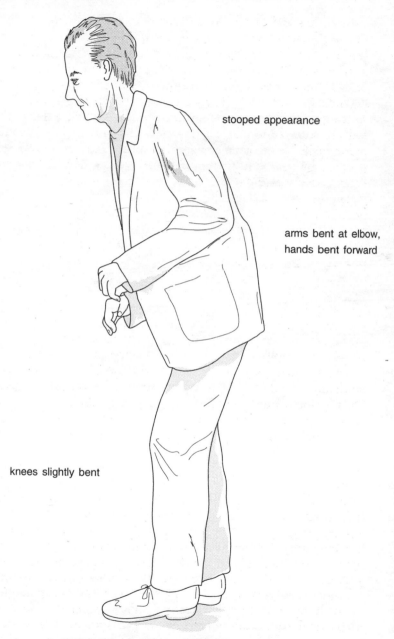

stooped appearance

arms bent at elbow,
hands bent forward

knees slightly bent

Standing posture in Parkinson's disease

problem in Parkinson's disease. The head and body do not move independently and spinning on the spot is virtually impossible. Thus, turning has to be accomplished as a whole-body manoeuvre, in which the body is moved round, like a statue, in a series of small steps.

The inco-ordination of gait also poses a problem in negotiating objects or narrow paths within the normal line of walking. The sudden appearance of these obstacles appears to interfere acutely with the normal rhythm of walking, so that people may freeze on the spot, engage in a series of small, unproductive steps (festination) or simply lose balance and fall over. For this reason, the house of a person with at least moderately advanced Parkinson's disease should be adapted to reduce unnecessary furniture, to place it out of the direct line of walking but within reach for support, to leave the doors open and preferably to widen the doorways. Climbing up and down stairs may be impossible for people with more advanced forms of the disorder and should be avoided because of the severe hazards of falling under those circumstances.

Loss of dexterity

Movements of the hands are markedly affected by the akinesia, particularly where careful or repetitive movements are required. Mild problems may produce difficulties in tasks such as fastening buttons, threading needles and counting change. With more advanced difficulties there are also problems in many of the normal activities associated with looking after yourself, including washing, dressing and eating. Writing tends to become smaller and more irregular. One classical type of writing abnormality in Parkinson's disease is writing that starts at normal size but then becomes progressively smaller, more compact and irregular as the person continues to write (micrographia).

Finger dexterity is one of the most sensitive aspects of movement to be affected by Parkinson's disease, so that even relatively minor forms of the condition may provoke significant difficulties in some of the finer but important activities of daily life. The inability to move fingers independently of the others can be a particularly telling sign of the presence of akinesia.

[Handwriting sample]

27/1/75
40 secs

14/1/76
25 secs

[Handwriting sample]

Sample of handwriting in Parkinson's disease

Tremor

The development of involuntary shaking of one part of the body is a particularly noticeable symptom to any patient or their relatives. Thus, people who develop tremor as a feature of Parkinson's disease tend to consult their doctor earlier than those who develop prominent akinesia or rigidity, merely because these latter symptoms creep on slowly and are not so immediately obvious. The tremor of Parkinson's disease typically occurs at rest and improves when the limb is in use, such as when holding an object.

The rest tremor usually affects the fingers, hands and head, but in more advanced cases the legs may be affected also. The main movement involved in this sort of tremor is synchronous opening and closing of the four fingers, combined with movements of the thumb and sometimes twisting of the wrist. The shaking has been termed a 'pill-rolling' tremor; this is because it resembles the movements made by old-fashioned pill-makers who moulded pills by rolling a paste-like substance containing the drugs between the thumb and forefinger of one hand. The tremor of Parkinson's disease may also affect the head, when it produces a nodding movement or a side-to-side shaking. Involuntary head movements of this kind are called titubation.

The Parkinsonian tremor usually occurs at a frequency of four to eight times per second; sometimes, however, a slightly different sort of tremor persists when the limb is in use and this tremor is often a little faster. The tremor of Parkinson's disease is increased by fear, anxiety or anger and sometimes by extreme joy. As with most involuntary movements, the tremor disappears in sleep.

Tremor is often more of a social embarrassment than a contributor to disability. Although many people with Parkinson's disease, or their relatives, think that the use of the hands is handicapped by the shaking, more often it is the accompanying akinesia or rigidity which is causing the difficulty.

Dyskinesia

The term dyskinesia refers to an abnormality of movement that is not directly due to Parkinson's disease but which can occur as a complication of treatment, usually treatment with the drug levodopa. The commonest form of dyskinesia is called chorea; this is quite unlike the rest tremor of Parkinson's disease. The involuntary movements of chorea are sometimes called semi-purposeful because they appear as if the person is about to begin some meaningful action but changes in mid-stream to undertake the beginning of another action, and so on in a disorderly fashion. This gives the general impression that the person is fidgety, twitchy or restless. In the face this may be evident as pulling faces, with raising and lowering of the eyebrows, movements of the eyes, opening and closing of the mouth and side-to-side movements of the jaw. The hands may open and close; the fingers rub against each other; and the body and legs move irregularly as if the person is sitting uncomfortably. In the more florid examples the head and neck may twist in brief writhing movements.

Rarely, the dyskinesias may take the form of more bizarre and sometimes violent shaking, particularly in patients who have been treated with levodopa for many years. More commonly, levodopa treatment may produce very brief twitching movements, usually of one arm or one leg, and often at night.

The relationship of these involuntary movements to levodopa treatment, and methods to resolve them, are discussed in Chapter 8.

Dystonia

Dystonia refers to an involuntary movement characterized by the apparent spasm of one set of muscles, deforming the limb into an abnormal posture. In Parkinson's disease this typically affects the legs; the foot may become twisted inwards so that the person feels that they are walking on the outside of the foot, this dystonia perhaps persisting for several minutes but sometimes much longer.

As with dyskinesias, the disorder is more common in patients treated with levodopa. Occasionally, however, dystonia of the foot, as described above, may occur as part of the disease itself. In patients treated with levodopa, the dystonias are often painful, and occur particularly in the early morning as the person rises from bed; dystonias that form part of the disease itself occur at any time of the day, and are usually painless and briefer than those caused by levodopa.

For treatment of this condition, see also Chapter 8.

6

Changes of memory and mood

Many books on Parkinson's disease do not make reference to problems with memory and mood because, for most people, they are not a major problem. However, we now recognize that difficulties with memory do occur in Parkinson's disease, and a proportion of people become depressed. Furthermore, some of the drugs that are used as treatment can affect memory and mood – sometimes for better, sometimes for worse. For those people who do have problems in this area it is important to recognize them and to find out their cause, because sometimes the problems may be connected with Parkinson's disease and sometimes they may be caused by something quite separate. In addition, it may be quite possible to help these symptoms by altering treatment. Even in the worst cases, understanding the problems can help us to come to terms with them.

So, for many people with Parkinson's disease, this chapter may not be important. We have included it, though, to help the proportion of people who do have difficulties in this area.

Memory

What causes memory problems?

We are all a bit sensitive about the idea that our intellectual faculties may fail – the last thing that most of us want is to become 'senile'. Many people also have the idea that 'senility', when it occurs, is somehow the fault of the person affected – perhaps they are feeble-minded, lacking in spirit or unable to stand up to the normal stresses of life. Many people think that 'senility', or dementia as it is often termed medically, is a special sort of mental illness, a sort of nervous breakdown. It is also easy to think that any form of memory disturbance, whether it be mild or severe, is inevitably the first step on the downward path to complete loss of independence. We easily assume that anyone with a memory problem must be suffering from senility, dementia or a speeding up of the aging process, and many people do not like to think of these problems because they find them distasteful. Until recently it has certainly never been the tradition of our society to tolerate this sort of problem.

But the truth is that dementia is caused as much by a disease of the brain as is Parkinson's disease. If you examine the brain of someone with Alzheimer's disease, the commonest cause of dementia, you will find obvious changes under the microscope that are as easily recognizable as the changes that occur in Parkinson's disease. People who develop dementia come from all walks of life. Dementia can strike the intellectually gifted as well as the mentally retarded. It affects people of strong character as well as those of nervous disposition. It occurs just as readily in those who have never had any psychiatric disease as in those who have required constant psychiatric care. It is only the way in which the disease manifests itself that people find difficult to accept or understand; and often they too readily assume that the behaviour is being conducted wilfully. So most of the common assumptions about dementia are untrue.

It is also untrue that any cause of memory disturbance inevitably leads to severe dementia. There are many, many causes of memory disturbance. Indeed, many of the causes of Parkinsonian syndrome listed in Chapter 1 can also produce memory problems, with or without the symptoms of Parkinson's disease. Some of these problems are mild while some of them are more severe; there is, however, a wide range. So it is possible to have a disease that produces mild impairment of memory without being part of the way down the road to complete dependence on other people. In fact, memory normally declines progressively with age. It is a common experience to find that your memory is less acute at 60 than it was at 30; this is such a normal experience that most tests of memory have built-in allowances for the age of the person. So when doctors assess complaints of memory they have to take account of the normal deterioration that occurs with age, and they have to recognize that there are many diseases that do produce impairment of memory, sometimes mildly but sometimes severely.

When memory problems are mild they usually amount to absent-mindedness – the sort of thing that happens to everybody on occasions, only a little more severely than normal. In such circumstances people may forget where they have put things; they forget appointments; they forget minor details of conversation, although they have no difficulty remembering the more important items. When they go shopping, they have to make a list because they cannot keep the items in their head.

Do not be alarmed if you experience these problems – they happen to everybody at some time or other. With true memory problems it is simply that they happen more often. However, if you are concerned that your memory is failing, you should certainly consult your doctor, who can then establish whether there is any cause for concern.

How common is memory loss in Parkinson's disease?

There are several different causes of memory loss in Parkinson's disease. As we have discussed, memory is not so sharp in older age anyway so people who develop Parkinson's disease later in life cannot expect to have such good memories. Parkinson's disease itself does produce an additional blunting of memory in many patients, even early in the disease, but this sort of memory problem is usually very mild and does not affect everyday life beyond a certain absent-mindedness. We do not know the cause of this mild memory loss, and it does not seem to be helped by levodopa or any of the dopaminergic drugs. Fortunately it is not usually a major problem.

Regrettably we have to accept the fact that serious loss of intellect (dementia) does occur with increasing age, so that sometimes such people are unkindly referred to as 'senile'. This condition affects perhaps one in 20 of the whole population aged over 65, but seems to be a little more common if you have Parkinson's disease as well; in addition to the normal relationship with age, perhaps an extra one person in ten will develop dementia specifically because they have Parkinson's disease. People who develop dementia tend to have a gradually worsening problem with memory and ability to cope with everyday life. In its most severe form they are unable to look after themselves and forget things over the course of a few minutes. They may even fail to recognize their own family. Sometimes there also seems to be a change of personality so that a person with a placid nature starts to become aggressive. They may have disturbance of sleep so that they tend to wander at night, and they may become lost, even in their own house. They may lose control of their urine and fail to eat unless prompted.

You should remember that the major risk of this condition stems from getting older, and not from Parkinson's disease – having Parkinson's disease merely increases the risk, and young people with Parkinson's disease seem hardly to develop these major problems at all.

Problems of memory loss

For the more elderly person, and the unlucky one who develops dementia, there can be problems with medication and mobility. Most of the drugs that are given for Parkinson's disease will make memory problems and confusion worse. Furthermore, anti-Parkinsonian drugs may provoke hallucinations when there is no dementia, but the risk is much greater in those people who do have dementia. This means that we sometimes have to compromise on treatment and forsake some of the mobility that the drugs will provide in order to reduce the side-effects of confusion. In addition, different drugs can be given to help the confusion itself. Care has to be taken, however, because, conversely, some of these drugs make the movement problems worse. Your doctor will advise you if you have a relative affected in this way.

Drugs for Parkinson's disease can interfere with memory even in people whose memory and intellect are normal. The anti-cholinergic drugs are particularly troublesome, so you should discuss this problem with your doctor if you are taking one of these drugs and you feel that your memory is poor.

Sometimes, poor memory can be caused directly by depression and will improve on antidepressant drugs.

Depression

What causes depression?

There are almost as many misconceptions about depression as

there are about dementia. Some people believe that depression only occurs in the weak-willed who cannot stand up to the stresses of life. Often they are advised to 'snap out of it'. But for the sufferer of severe depression this is unkind advice; the person is usually quite unable to 'snap out of it' – and it was not their wish to be in that state in the first place. It is also often assumed that depression is always caused by something unpleasant in life. These are, however, half truths at most.

Depression is now believed to comprise at least two types. One is undoubtedly, and often quite understandably, caused by a reaction to something unpleasant in life. Thus it is commonplace to become depressed after the death of a close relative; it is also frequent for depression to develop in the context of an unhappy marriage. Not surprisingly, people with physical disability, who are not able to do as much as they used to, become depressed if they cannot adapt to their new circumstances.

But there is another sort of depression. Sometimes the depression arises 'out of the blue' in someone who seemingly has a perfectly happy life. This form of depression is sometimes called endogenous or biological, because it is believed to be caused by chemical changes occurring within the brain; in the same way that chemical changes in certain parts of the brain can cause the movement difficulties of Parkinson's disease, so can chemical changes in other parts of the brain produce depression. The features of this sort of depression may be very much those of the first sort except that there is no obvious cause for it. Thus we often hear people say 'I cannot understand why he is depressed because he has everything going so well for him.' Such a person may be suffering from the effects of chemical change in the brain.

How common is depression in Parkinson's disease?

Depression is common in Parkinson's disease; it occurs in the early as well as in the later stages, although the causes may be different.

Perhaps as many as one in five of people with Parkinson's disease have depression about the time of diagnosis. Sometimes this is caused by the shock of the news that they have Parkinson's disease, but part of it may also be due to chemical changes in parts of the brain other than the basal ganglia. This form of depression often improves when treatment is begun. Depression also occurs in people who have had Parkinson's disease for a number of years. Again, this may be a psychological reaction to the failure of the drugs to work so well; however, it also occurs for no obvious reason, and we believe that this situation arises as a result of a change in the brain chemistry.

Problems of depression

It is important to recognize the existence of depression because it can be confused with other symptoms of Parkinson's disease. Depression produces a loss of initiative and drive – the get up and go. It can produce general feelings of weakness and tiredness. Depression also reduces appetite and may lead to weight loss. Constipation may occur. Sleep can be disrupted, so that depressed people tend to wake in the early hours of the morning and have difficulty in returning to sleep. Many depressed people also complain of general aches and pains and difficulty in coping with life.

Many of these symptoms are also typical features of Parkinson's disease without depression, and will not be put down to depression unless this is considered. It is particularly important to bear this possibility in mind, because depression does not necessarily produce a feeling of sadness; someone can be depressed without realizing it. Depression should be considered if there is little or no improvement when the anti-Parkinsonian drugs are adjusted. Treatment with a different sort of medication, antidepressant drugs, can relieve many of these physical symptoms if they are caused by depression.

Do any other mental problems occur?

Many people use the term memory to refer to all the intellectual activities that they carry out. Strictly speaking, though, memory merely refers to the ability to hold facts in your head for anything from seconds to years. The more complex functions of the brain involve more than just memory. For example, we use our brain when we attend to something, such as listening to a television programme, but we do not have to remember it. There are special functions of the brain that allow us to make judgments and decisions – what we will have for breakfast, whether we can afford a new coat, who to vote for. Other functions of the brain allow us to be more or less adaptable – a person playing in a football team, for example, has to be particularly skilful at altering his approach when the game seems to be changing its pattern, changing his attitude rapidly so that he adapts readily to the new situation. Special mechanisms of the brain are involved in planning our future, whether this be for the next few hours or the next few years: we plan our week's activities; we plan our savings for some future event; we plan next year's holiday and the build-up to it; teachers may plan out a lesson in detail. All of these functions involve complex activities of the brain, but they need not involve memory. They are, however, just as important.

People who suffer from dementia, as well as suffering from memory loss, also have problems in these complex activities of the brain. In fact it is difficulties with these functions that cause most of their problems of everyday life, including their inability to organize their day, to make sensible judgments and to plan for the future. It is not surprising, then, that when a patient with Parkinson's disease also suffers from dementia it is sometimes difficult to be sure what is the main cause of their everyday problems. The demented Parkinsonian patient may have had Parkinson's disease for a number of years and show considerable loss of mobility. In these circumstances it is very easy to assume that someone's difficulty in coping is due entirely to their problems in getting about; but if the person also suffers from dementia – even mild dementia – then their difficulties in carrying out the tasks of everyday life will be just as much a result of their loss of judgment, planning, attention and adaptation as of their physical difficulty in carrying out tasks.

We often fight shy of thinking that a close relative, say, who has Parkinson's disease, might be showing signs of dementia. However we should be prepared to consider this possibility, especially if their difficulty in coping seems to be more than can be explained merely by a difficulty with movement. And, of course, the same situation can arise with depression. So if you have a relative who is not coping as well as you expect you should discuss with your doctor the possibility that they may be depressed or showing early signs of dementia. As we have discussed the situation is not hopeless, because depression can be treated and the other mental effects can often be helped by adjustment of medication.

As with memory, the brain functions of planning, adaptation and judgment do tend to get a little worse as we get older. In addition, research has shown that people with Parkinson's disease may have mild additional problems in these areas. This does not mean that, if you have Parkinson's disease, you are going to become demented. Most people do not do so, even though we can often pick up a slight loss of ability in these areas, using tests similar to IQ tests. More often than not you would not notice any problem in your everyday life. Sometimes the slight loss of adaptability, judgment and planning can show itself as a loss of concentration or an unwillingness to adapt to new situations. But it may be friends or relatives who notice this more than the individual with Parkinson's disease; this is because none of us is inclined to look critically at ourselves and we are usually unwilling to admit that we do not readily adapt to change.

These complex activities of the brain do not seem to be linked to the dopamine-containing cells of the basal ganglia, and treatment with levodopa does not usually improve them. Instead these mental activities seem to depend more on the frontal lobes, situated in the front part of the brain, more or less behind the forehead and between the temples. Research has shown that in Parkinson's disease this part of the brain is not working quite as well as we would expect but, at the moment, we are not sure why this happens. You should realize, however, that this is seldom a serious problem, except for the unfortunate few who become demented.

One particular mental difficulty that has been specially linked with Parkinson's disease is called bradyphrenia, slowness of thinking. It is not the same as the other problems that we have mentioned, and it is not the same as dementia – it does not affect judgment, planning or adaptability. Bradyphrenia has been used to describe a certain slowness of response, for example in reply to a question; you may simply have to wait a second or two longer, but the answer is perfectly sensible when it is produced. Bradyphrenia may be linked to depression because depression can produce the same kind of slowness.

When dealing with Parkinson's disease it is important to recognize mental difficulties when they occur, and not to blame everything on the problems with movement. Most people with this sort of mental difficulty are not behaving in that way on purpose – they simply may not be able to produce an answer quickly, to show initiative and drive, or to be as adaptable, happy and carefree as they used to be. Indeed, they are no more able to perform these functions properly than they are able to use their muscles properly. Morever, they often do not appreciate that they are experiencing mental problems at all and will not respond to exhortations that they 'should realize how difficult' they have become.

However, you have to get the balance right. This chapter has drawn attention to some of the mental problems that can occur in Parkinson's disease, both because it helps if you can understand them and because treatment can be offered in some circumstances. You should therefore try to recognize these problems when they are present. But remember that many people with Parkinon's disease do not suffer from these problems; if you or someone you know has Parkinson's disease you must be careful not to think of yourself or them as feeble-minded. Many people who do not understand Parkinson's disease are all too ready to blame a patient's difficulty in coping on some kind of mental problem. And it is just as easy to blame the problems in movement on some mental difficulty as it is to ignore the mental problems and to put all the day-to-day difficulties down to problems in getting about or simple bloody-mindedness. Try to keep an open mind, and ask your doctor if you have particular worries.

7

Other possible complaints

This chapter describes some symptoms of Parkinson's disease that cannot easily be attributed to the difficulty in movement or to the psychological features of the disease. They are all common in Parkinson's disease; however, they also occur in other conditions and you should be careful not to blame every symptom you have upon your Parkinson's disease. It is usually best to ask your doctor, because many other conditions can cause similar symptoms. They may require special tests or a different sort of treatment.

Constipation

Constipation is a common symptom in the elderly, but it is more common if you also have Parkinson's disease. It is primarily caused because the muscles that move the bowels become rather sluggish, but it can also be caused by some of the drug treatments, particularly anticholinergic drugs such as benzhexol (Artane, see Chapter 8).

Constipation, by itself, is not a serious problem. Many people worry if they do not open their bowels each day, but you will not do yourself any harm as long as you are not developing other symptoms, such as stomach pains or alternating diarrhoea and constipation. Failure to open the bowels every day will not affect your Parkinson's disease or lead to some sort of poisoning. But you should check with your doctor that your constipation is due to your Parkinson's disease, particularly if it has developed recently without any change of treatment.

If the constipation is due to the Parkinson's disease there are several things you can do.

- Try to eat a diet that is rich in roughage, such as fresh fruit, vegetables and salad.
- Add two tablespoons of wheat bran to your breakfast cereal, and try to take extra bran at other times of the day. Bran tablets are also available.
- Drink at least half a litre of water each day in addition to your usual drinks; try not to let yourself get too thirsty.
- Do not use laxatives regularly because, after a time, these make the bowels more sluggish.
- Take regular exercise, such as a 30-minute walk each morning, if you can manage it.

If the constipation persists, despite these measures, then you can obtain glycerine suppositories or small doses of laxatives, preferably from your doctor.

Difficulty in passing water

Parkinson's disease can cause various problems in passing water. These include slowness in starting, dribbling for some time afterwards, passing urine more frequently and difficulty in holding your water. These symptoms are caused by difficulty in co-ordinating the muscles that control the opening and closing of the bladder. In addition, some of the drugs, particularly the anticholinergic drugs, may produce difficulty in starting, and dribbling afterwards.

But, again, there are many other causes of these problems, particularly in the elderly. Infections of the urine are common, particularly in women – they are easily diagnosed and treated with antibiotics. In men, enlargement of the prostate gland can produce very similar symptoms; the problem can be treated by a minor procedure or an operation if necessary. In women, mild degrees of prolapse of the uterus (womb) or weakness of the wall of the bladder often occur after giving birth to children; again this problem has nothing to do with Parkinson's disease and can be cured by a gynaecological operation. So if you have these symptoms you should consult your doctor before blaming them on the Parkinson's disease.

Sexual problems

Most people are shy about discussing sexual difficulties, but they can be a real problem in Parkinson's disease. Many people, with or without Parkinson's disease, find their sexual appetite waning with age in any case, and this is no cause for concern. Some people with Parkinson's disease have an active sexual appetite, but are put off because of the physical difficulties of their condition. Often sexual problems arise more from a fear of failure than from real physical handicap. The presence of depression can also seriously interfere with sexual drive and performance, but this will improve on treatment of the depression.

Some of the drugs used in Parkinson's disease, particularly anticholinergic drugs, can interfere with a man's ability to achieve erections. There are, however, other causes of erectile failure, such as diabetes, so you should consult your doctor if this is a problem for you. In men, failure to achieve erections is often caused by anxiety, but you should not assume this without a medical opinion. If you find that you are having normal erections in your sleep or on awakening in the morning, but not during attempted sexual activity, the problem is more likely to be due to stress than a purely physical problem.

Soon after levopoda was produced it was said that it had an aphrodisiac effect, increasing sexual drive and performance. There may well be a few people for whom this is true, and you should consider this possibility if you have recently started on treatment and noticed a marked change in your sexual drive. More often than not, however, people do not experience any change in sexual drive from levodopa alone, except for the natural sense of well-being that comes with greater physical ability.

For the minority who do suffer from failure to achieve erections that cannot be dealt with by any other means, there are ways of helping you to engage in normal sexual activities. Mechanical aids and other treatments can be used to support the penis during sexual intercourse or to produce an erection if this does not occur naturally. Some of the new drug treatments to help erectile difficulties include sildenafil (Viagra) and apomorphine (in lower doses than used to treat movement problems in Parkinson's Disease; see Chapter 8). You can obtain further advice on sexual difficulties from your doctor, a specialist hospital clinic, or the organization SPOD (Sexual Problems of the Disabled).

Sweating

Changes in sweating occur in Parkinson's disease. Sometimes these consist of reduced sweating in response to heat, but other people have episodes of excessive sweating, the latter occurring most often in people who have response fluctuations to treatment, such as the on/off phenomenon (see Chapter 8). Sweating may occur because of the muscular activity that occurs during severe dyskinesia (abnormality of movement, see page 42); however, some people seem to develop their sweating bouts during periods of akinesia (slowness of movement, see page 34) when they are least active.

The reasons for these sweating changes are uncertain but they can be very severe, sometimes producing drenching of the bedclothes at night. The relationship to treatment is often unpredictable. Excessive sweating is often helped by levodopa therapy, but a change to a depamine agonist (see Chapter 8) may be helpful if the sweating occurs during treatment with levodopa. In other cases, the drug propranolol may be helpful.

Salivation

Parkinson's disease sometimes causes problems with salivation; saliva tends to collect in the mouth and drool from the corners. This problem may be due to difficulty in the normal swallowing of saliva, but some patients with Parkinson's disease also seem to produce excessive saliva.

Some of the anti-Parkinsonian drugs, particularly the anti-cholinergic drugs, can dry the mouth as a side-effect and can be useful to help this symptom. One of them, hyoscine can be given as a skin patch to provide relief for most of the day or night.

Dizziness

The commonest cause of severe dizziness in Parkinson's disease is a fall in blood pressure on standing.

When we stand up, there is a natural tendency for the blood pressure to fall because blood collects in the veins of the legs. We have a set of reflexes that rapidly come into action to correct this fall in blood pressure, but in Parkinson's disease these reflexes may be sluggish. The problem is worse on standing rapidly, or on prolonged standing in one place. The symptoms will also be worse in a hot environment, after meals, or on rising during the night, for example to visit the toilet. People who have dizziness on standing should be particularly careful under these circumstances; they should sit on the edge of the bed for one or two minutes before standing, and should stand from a chair rather slowly. They should avoid standing for long periods in one place or, if they have to do so, should regularly transfer the weight from foot to foot.

The drugs levodopa, and the dopamine agonists (see Chapter 8) may make this symptom worse, or even produce it for the first time. Anticholinergic drugs do not seem to affect the symptom. For many people the development of this dizziness limits the dose of drugs which they can take. If the problem is brought on by drugs, it always goes away when the dose is reduced or the drug is changed to another type. In addition, some of the drugs will produce the symptom when they are first begun, but people then get used to the drugs and the symptom disappears. So it is worth trying to continue with a prescribed drug even if it produces side-effects in the early stages unless, of course, these are particularly unpleasant.

For people who do have a fall in blood pressure on standing, which is not helped by adjustment of drug dosage, the symptoms can be controlled by raising the head of the bed three to four inches at night, by the wearing of elastic stockings to support the veins of the legs and by taking frequent strong coffee. Drugs can also be prescribed by your doctor that will increase the blood pressure.

Less severe forms of dizziness – usually vague lightheadedness – are also common in Parkinson's disease. This form of dizziness is not usually due to change in blood pressure, and occurs whether the person is sitting or standing. It is a symptom with many causes, including depression and side-effects of drugs.

Some of the medicines normally used for the treatment of dizziness can make your Parkinson's disease temporarily worse. One of the more common ones is prochlorperazine (Stemetil). If you have Parkinson's disease and develop dizziness, you should be cautious of taking this drug; you would do better to ask your doctor for another one, if possible.

Ankle swelling

Ankle swelling can occur in Parkinson's disease, usually getting worse as the day goes on.

Normally fluid in the legs is pushed upwards, back to the heart, by the pumping action of the muscles in the legs acting on the veins. In Parkinson's disease, however, these muscles do not work so well, so the fluid tends to collect around the ankles. The problem is more common if you spend long periods of time sitting in a chair, and is helped by walking about. It can be further helped by putting your feet up on a stool whenever you sit down and by the wearing of elastic support stockings. Sometimes you may need to take water pills to remove the fluid, but you should be careful with these because they can cause your blood pressure to drop and so produce dizziness, and can also increase your constipation.

Swelling of the ankles can occasionally be caused from the anti-Parkinsonian treatments, particularly amantadine and dopamine agonists (see Chapter 8).

Trouble with the eyes

Many patients with Parkinson's disease complain of not being able to see clearly. Part of the problem is probably linked directly with Parkinson's disease, although the exact reason is uncertain. This area of difficulty seems to affect particularly the ability to judge distances or to make out clearly the shape of objects.

More commonly, though, simple blurring of vision is caused by the drug treatment, particularly the anticholinergic drugs such as benzhexol (Artane). This drug partially paralyses the muscles within the eye which are used to focus the eye on close objects. Blurring of vision caused by anticholinergic drugs therefore usually affects close vision, such as reading, sewing or writing. Anticholinergic drugs should not be used in people who have a particular sort of eye disease known as closed angle glaucoma.

Occasionally, people with Parkinson's disease have difficulty in keeping their eyes open; the eyelids seem to close of their own accord and for no very good reason. The symptoms occur without any feelings of tiredness or desire to sleep. This symptom has been called apraxia of lid opening. In other cases there can be a forcible spasm of the muscles of the eyes, which has been called blepharospasm. This condition usually occurs in

Parkinsonian syndromes, as distinct from true Parkinson's disease (see Chapter 1), but it can be made worse or better by anti-Parkinsonian drugs. Completely different drug treatments are also available for this sort of problem, and nowadays this sort of eye spasm can be helped by injection of a paralysing drug (botulinum toxin) into the muscles around the eye. These injections can relieve the spasm for two to three months and they do not affect muscles in other parts of the body.

Everybody blinks their eyes regularly, several times each minute, but this blinking occurs less frequently in Parkinson's disease. The reduction in blinking tends to produce a staring expression of the eyes, and may sometimes lead to irritation of the eyes because they are wiped by the eyelids less often than normal.

Greasy skin

Parkinson's disease may cause greasiness of the skin. This is because there is overactivity of the sebaceous glands that produce the waxy sheen over the skin. It is more common with the post-encephalitic form of Parkinsonism.

Breathing difficulties

People with Parkinson's disease may become breathless because of the extra effort required to carry out activity. In addition, the muscles of the chest tend to be stiffer and move less readily in Parkinson's disease, problems similar to those affecting the muscles of the arms and legs. Because the chest muscles are important for normal breathing, it is easy to understand how such breathlessness can occur when these muscles are affected.

But it would certainly be wrong to ascribe all such breathlessness to Parkinson's disease without further investigation. If you do become breathless you should see your doctor, who will undoubtedly want to examine your chest and heart. And if you do have a chest or heart condition, then some of the drugs used for the treatment of Parkinson's disease, such as levodopa, may make the problem worse. The difficulty can often be solved by adjustment of Parkinsonian drugs or by specific treatment of your chest or heart condition.

8

Medicines used in Parkinson's disease

Can I be cured?

One of the first things that people want to know when they have been told that they have Parkinson's disease is what can be done about it. Since the 1960s enormous advances have been made in the treatment of Parkinson's disease, such that very helpful medicines now exist that can alleviate the problems of the majority of patients.

However the treatment involves taking medicine on a day-to-day basis, possibly for ever; this is because the medicines effectively put right the chemical changes that occur in the brain (see Chapter 3). The treatment is not therefore a cure, in the sense that a course of tablets will get rid of the disorder permanently, like a course of antibiotics for pneumonia. Nevertheless, the help that is now available for the Parkinsonian sufferer is vastly greater than it was as recently as the early 1960s.

A 63-year-old man was referred to me by his general practitioner because he complained of difficulty in walking and problems with writing and fastening buttons. For some time he had been thought to have arthritis, but had not improved on anti-arthritic drugs. His general practitioner suspected a diagnosis of Parkinson's disease because he found akinesia of finger movements, cog-wheel rigidity in both arms and a stooped gait with small steps. There was also a slight tremor of the right hand at rest.

In the referral, his general practitioner pointed out that he suspected Parkinson's disease but asked me if I would confirm the diagnosis. In the meantime, he had begun treatment with Madopar (levodopa), 65.2 mg, twice daily. By the time of his arrival at the outpatient clinic the dose had been increased to 125 mg, twice daily, and the patient had become completely symptom-free; his walking had returned to normal and he was able to perform all movements of his hands without difficulty.

I examined the man and found no signs of Parkinson's disease. I reported to the general practitioner that there was no trace of Parkinson's disease but I suspected that the signs had been eliminated by his successful treatment. Because the diagnosis was so important, I asked the patient to cut his dose of Madopar in half and to return one week later. At that time there were clear signs of Parkinson's disease and his symptoms had returned. We established the diagnosis of Parkinson's disease and returned his treatment to the higher level.

This demonstrates how, in some cases, the treatment of Parkinson's disease can alter the situation so that no one, including a doctor, would know that you had the condition.

Do I have to take treatment?

Although the prescribed drugs will help whatever problems of Parkinson's disease you may have, as long as you keep taking the medication, there is no absolute need for you to take this treatment. Indeed, some people with Parkinson's disease have only mild problems that do not interfere with their everyday life, and often prefer to carry on as they are without taking tablets each day.

Unfortunately Parkinson's disease does tend to get worse with time, and beginning the treatment early in the progression of the disease does not seem to limit this progression. What doctors tend to do now is to introduce drug treatment when they and the patient feel it is necessary, and to use the lowest dose of drugs concomitant with each person's individual needs. Obviously these needs will vary a lot, between for example someone who is relatively inactive and someone who is, say, a concert pianist and needs excellent co-ordination to carry out their job. In addition, drugs have side-effects in some people in the short or long term, and these considerations must be balanced against the benefits that the drugs provide. However, if you feel that you do need treatment you should not be frightened of taking it; it can be very helpful, and your doctor will be keeping a close eye on you to make sure that there are no problems.

This rule – that the treatment is not a cure – applies to the vast majority of drugs used for the treatment of Parkinson's disease, but there is one exception. The drug selegiline has been in use for some time to help some of the response fluctuations that occur later in the disease. Recently, however, doctors from the United States have reported that the drug may slow down the progression of the disease; they discovered that patients who started on selegiline when their condition was first diagnosed continued for a longer period before needing levodopa treatment than did patients who did not take selegiline. This does not necessarily mean that selegiline slows down the natural progression of the disease, because a similar effect would occur if selegiline merely had some beneficial effect on the symptoms of the disease, without affecting its natural speed of progression. Selegiline does indeed seem to have just such an effect, but not all the findings of the American doctors can be explained in this way.

The patients in the American study have now been followed up for a longer period and the early beneficial effects of selegiline do not seem so great. Also, a more recent study from the United Kingdom examined the effects of selegiline on the progression of Parkinson's disease and found that it did not slow down progression of the condition at all. In fact, the death rate over the years in those patients that were taking selegiline together with levodopa was actually higher than in those patients who were taking levodopa alone. We do not know the explanation for this finding and why it differs from that in the American study. Some doctors in Britain are now recommending that their patients stop treatment with selegiline until the findings of the British study are explained. However, we have found that some patients seem to need their selegiline; they deteriorated quite a lot when the drug was withdrawn and had to be put back on it. Do not be alarmed if you are taking selegiline – we are not treating it as a dangerous drug but we are still trying to find out the explanation for the results of the British research and why it differs from that in the United States. A lot of research in medicine yields controversial results and it is only by continuing the research that we can obtain a more definite answer that will allow us to offer the best treatment to our patients.

Which drug should I take?

Some people tend to compare the treatment that they have received from their doctor with the treatment received by another person from another doctor. Although it is important that you seek the best treatment, you should be careful not to compare yourself too closely with someone else. The problems experienced by different people with Parkinson's disease vary quite considerably, and the drugs used for these various problems differ correspondingly. In addition, some people develop side-effects on drugs that do not affect others. Thus, treatment that is suitable for one person may be quite unsuitable for another.

If you are concerned about your treatment you should discuss it quite openly with your doctor, mentioning the particular points that concern you most.

How often do I need to take treatment?

All drugs differ according to the number of times per day that they need to be taken; some can be given only once or twice a day, others need to be given much more frequently. One reason for these differences is that the drugs differ in the rate at which the body clears them from the bloodstream. In Parkinson's disease this principle is even more complicated because the frequency of tablet-taking must be varied a great deal according to the particular problems of the individual. Some people who have marked fluctuations (see below) may be taking tablets very frequently, even every hour or two; other people, who do not have the same problems, may need to take the same drug only two or three times per day.

Although you and your doctor should strive to achieve the simplest possible timetable of treatment, you should try to stick rigidly to the timing of your medications because this is often very important in the effective management of Parkinson's disease.

Do all drugs have the same effects?

Many people wonder why they are taking more than one drug if they are all directed at correcting the same chemical imbalance within the brain (see Chapter 3). However, this idea about the way in which drugs act in Parkinson's disease is not quite accurate. In fact different drugs have slightly different effects on the brain chemistry, and can be of varying benefit for the different problems of Parkinson's disease. For example, some drugs may be more helpful for the akinesia, whereas other drugs appear better for dealing with tremor. In addition, some drugs, such as selegiline and entacapone, are used not as a main treatment but to support the action of other drugs, such as levodopa. People who have a variety of problems may therefore find themselves on a mixture of drugs.

Drugs used in Parkinson's disease

Anticholinergics

The anticholinergics include a number of drugs that all act in a similar way, that is by blocking the action of one of the brain chemicals, acetylcholine. Although it is known that the main problem in Parkinson's disease is caused by loss of another chemical, dopamine, it was thought at one time that the problems were due specifically to an alteration of the balance between the two chemicals, acetylcholine and dopamine. Thus, normal function could be restored either by replacing dopamine or by blocking the action of acetylcholine. Charcot, who suggested naming Parkinson's disease after James Parkinson, in fact used an anticholinergic drug in the 19th century but the main use of anticholinergics began around the 1940s and 1950s, prior to the development of levodopa treatment.

Anticholinergics have only a mild to moderate effect on the symptoms of Parkinson's disease, producing approximately 25 per cent improvement on average. The main signs of Parkinson's

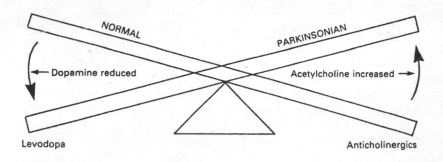

Action of anticholinergic drugs

disease – tremor, rigidity and akinesia – are helped approximately equally, but problems with balance and walking tend to be helped much less. Anticholinergic treatment is certainly not as effective as levodopa treatment, and tends to be used as a first-line therapy only for mild early cases. Some doctors believe that anticholinergics have a particularly good effect on tremor and use them in combination with levodopa; however, this is certainly not a universal rule and the risk of side-effects of combined treatment is greater than that of using one drug alone.

The main anticholinergic drugs are:

- benzhexol (Artane)
- orphenadrine (Dispal)
- benztropine (Cogentin)
- procyclidine (Kemadrin)
- and methixene (Tremonil)

Many patients are unable to take large doses of anticholinergics because of the side-effects. These include dry mouth, blurring of vision, difficulty in passing urine, constipation, dizziness, confusion, insomnia, sedation, impotence, poor memory and agitation. The anticholinergic drugs should not be taken by anyone who has narrow-angle glaucoma, while the side-effects of memory loss and confusion occur particularly in more elderly patients or those with the memory loss of Parkinson's disease (see Chapter 6).

Anticholinergics may be particularly helpful in people who produce a lot of saliva, because of the effects they have on drying the mouth. One anticholinergic drug, hyoscine, can be given through a skin patch and is helpful in dealing with the problem of excess salivation.

Amantadine

The effect of amantadine on Parkinson's disease was discovered accidentally. The drug was first introduced for the treatment of virus diseases, although it subsequently proved to be largely ineffective in this respect. However in 1968 the drug was given to a Parkinsonian patient for the treatment of influenza, and there was a noticeable improvement in his Parkinsonian symptoms. Since then the drug has been used under very similar circumstances to those of anticholinergics. Thus, it is used in patients with mild disease, and sometimes in those with predominant tremor. The effect of the drug used alone is relatively slight, but it can also be useful as an addition to levodopa treatment. Side-effects are relatively few and consist of mild agitation, sleeplessness, swelling of the ankles and skin rashes. Sometimes, confusions and hallucinations may develop when the drug is used in combination with levodopa. Recently, amantadine has also been shown to suppress dyskinesias, independent of its anti-Parkinsonian effect.

Levodopa

The discovery that the main problem in Parkinson's disease was the lack of the chemical dopamine led to attempts to treat Parkinson's disease by replacing the missing chemical. It is not possible for dopamine to pass into the brain from the bloodstream, but the problem is solved by using levodopa. Levodopa can be taken by mouth, passes from the bloodstream into the brain, then once in the brain is converted to dopamine – the active chemical.

When levodopa was first used for the treatment of Parkinson's disease in the early 1960s the effects were dramatic. Many people who had suffered considerable disability from the disease were suddenly 'switched on', as it were, when levodopa was administered. Since then, levodopa treatment in one form or

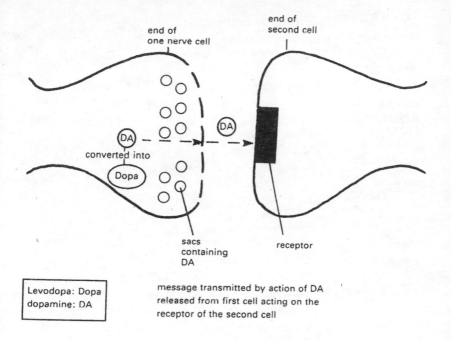

message transmitted by action of DA
released from first cell acting on the
receptor of the second cell

Levodopa: Dopa
dopamine: DA

Action of levodopa

another has been in the forefront of treatment for Parkinson's disease.

Some of the early attempts to use levodopa were limited by the side-effects of nausea and vomiting, but this problem has been much improved in the newer drugs, Madopar and Sinemet. In both of these preparations levodopa is mixed with another drug that blocks many of the side-effects of levodopa without interfering with its main action in the brain. These two preparations differ only in the drug that blocks the levodopa side-effects; in theory, there is practically nothing to choose between them, but some patients seem to have better control of their symptoms, and fewer side-effects, on one rather than the other.

Sinemet is prescribed as Sinemet 110 and Sinemet 275, which differ in the dose of levodopa. Sinemet Plus is equivalent to Sinemet 110 but has more of the drug to block side-effects. Sinemet LS is equivalent to half-strength Sinemet Plus. Madopar is prescribed as capsules, Madopar 62.5, Madopar 125 and

Madopar 250, which differ in the dose of levodopa. In addition two other types of preparation of levodopa are available.

Madopar Dispersible is a preparation that can be suspended in water; this is particularly helpful for people who have difficulty swallowing tablets or capsules. In addition, the medication reaches the bloodstream rather faster than ordinary Madopar, so is useful in providing a 'kick start' in the mornings or during 'off' periods. Madopar CR (CR stands for controlled release) is a slow release preparation of Madopar that delivers the drug to the bloodstream at a much slower, steadier rate than ordinary Madopar, so that its effects last longer and fluctuate less. This preparation can help those patients who have marked fluctuations in control (see below). However, the effective dose of Madopar CR is different from ordinary Madopar; in changing from Madopar to Madopar CR the dose will need to be increased, on average, by 50 per cent.

Madopar Dispersible is available in tablets of strength 62.5 or 125 mg. Madopar CR is available as 125-mg capsules. A slow release form of Sinemet (Sinemet CR) is also available and has similar benefits to Madopar CR in delivering the drug more slowly into the bloodstream. Sinemet CR is available in tablets of strength 250 mg and also as half-strength 125-mg tablets known as Half Sinemet CR.

A common side-effect of levodopa is nausea or vomiting, particularly during the early stages of treatment, but many people find that these side-effects wear off with time. Levodopa also causes the blood pressure to fall on standing, so that you may experience dizziness on standing. If so you should consult your doctor to have your standing blood pressure checked.

Mental changes are common side-effects of levodopa, particularly in the elderly; these include nightmares, sleep disturbance and, in more severe cases, confusion and hallucinations. Occasionally this can be a very alarming experience. However, unless there is any underlying mental impairment from the disease, it always improves as the dosage of levodopa is reduced, even though this reduction may make the problems with movement worse. In patients with more advanced disease, who suffer a combination of severe movement problems and dementia, one has to compromise on a dose of drugs that produces the best effect on the physical disability without making the mental disability worse.

Rare side-effects are alteration of heart rhythm, discoloration of urine, sweating and allergies. The side-effects of dyskinesia are discussed below, as well as in Chapter 5.

A 74-year-old lady had had Parkinson's disease for eight years. She had been managing well but, over the previous year, she had begun to notice that each dose of treatment seemed to wear off before the next one was due. Her treatment, which had been managed by her general practitioner, consisted of Sinemet 275 three times daily. At first her treatment was altered to Sinemet 110 seven times daily. Although this reduced the end-of-dose deterioration, she found that she was becoming generally stiff and immobile as the day progressed. The dose of drugs was therefore increased to Sinemet 110, nine, and then ten, times daily.

On reaching the higher dose she became severely confused. She believed that her daughter, with whom she had lived for the last ten years, was threatening to kill her and she repeatedly telephoned the police to complain of this. She displayed severe agitation and spent large parts of the day and night wandering around the house in anguish. She also complained repeatedly of 'wasps' and 'helicopters' that seemed to fly through the room without warning. When her daughter failed to remove these imaginary objects the patient became even more agitated.

She was admitted acutely to hospital and the dose of Sinemet was adjusted, ultimately to 110 eight times daily. All confusion and hallucinations ceased and, with adjustment of timing, her mobility was satisfactory, except for the evening when she was habitually inactive anyway.

Levodopa treatment has a dramatic effect on most Parkinsonian symptoms, particularly in the early stages, although tremor responds less well than akinesia or rigidity. Since akinesia has the most disabling effect on the activities of daily life, levodopa can restore normal functioning and indeed completely abolish all the signs of Parkinson's disease. In the early stages of the disease virtually everyone will respond if they are able to tolerate reasonable doses of the drug. Indeed, doctors usually reconsider the diagnosis if patients fail to respond to this drug.

The best dose of levodopa differs from one person to the next.

However, when the drug is first started, there may be a delay of days or even weeks before the maximal benefit is achieved, so weeks or months may be required before the best dose is found. Treatment is usually begun with a small dose twice or three times daily. In mild disease each dose will carry the patient over until the next dose, so they will notice little variation in the effect of the drug through the day.

If the dose of levodopa is too high you may develop dyskinesias – involuntary movements produced by the levodopa, and described in Chapter 5. Sometimes these dyskinesias occur transiently about 30 minutes or so after each dose, when the levels of the drug in the bloodstream reach their highest level. This problem usually responds to a small reduction in the size of each dose, taking a little less drug more frequently or changing to the controlled release preparation of Madopar or Sinemet. On other occasions the dyskinesias are persistent throughout the day. Often, this is a reflection of too high a total daily dose, and usually responds to a reduction in dosage.

Some patients experience perfect control of their Parkinson's disease with little change of dose over many years. Others find that the condition gradually deteriorates but they are able to maintain near perfect control by slight increases in the dose of drugs. Unfortunately, a proportion of patients do develop problems in control of their disease after approximately seven or more years of treatment with levodopa. Since most people who have had Parkinson's disease for this length of time will have been treated with levodopa, it is difficult for doctors to be sure whether the problems stem from simple progression of the disease or from the effects of long-term treatment with levodopa. Regardless of the origin, these patients begin to develop noticeable fluctuations in the control of their Parkinson's disease through the day. These problems fall into various patterns.

End-of-dose deterioration is caused by a reduction in the duration of effect of each dose of drug. When there are, for example, six hours between each dose, benefit may be achieved for the first, say, two hours. Thereafter the drug seems to wear off so that the person is left with four hours of akinesia until the next dose is taken. This problem can be helped by taking smaller doses of the drug more frequently, by the use of controlled release Madopar or Sinemet or by the addition of selegiline or entacapone (see below). Drugs known as dopamine agonists, such as pergolide or labergoline (discussed below), can also be used as an additional or substitute treatment for levodopa in these circumstances, as each dose of pergolide or labergoline tends to last longer than an equivalent dose of levodopa.

Peak-dose dyskinesia often accompanies end-of-dose deterioration. After each dose of levodopa, the blood level of the drug rises until it reaches a peak about 30 minutes later. At this point, dyskinesias develop and persist for a further 15–30 minutes. Although this phenomenon can occur early in the disease when the doses are too high, it occurs more readily, and at lower doses, later in the disease.

End-of-dose dyskinesia refers to dyskinesia developing as the blood level of levodopa is falling, so it tends to occur during the wearing-off period. The reason for this is not known.

Early morning benefit occurs in a small proportion of patients. Soon after rising in the morning they experience a brief period of freedom from Parkinsonian symptoms, even without medication. Although less dramatic than this, many more patients find the morning to be relatively free, the problems of movement increasing gradually through the rest of the day.

With the more advanced forms of the disease, the changes in mobility can take place very quickly, sometimes over a matter of a few seconds; one minute a person may be able to get about quite normally, although often with dyskinesias, but the next they have become quite immobile and helpless. The speed of change can be so dramatic that people with this condition may feel as if a switch is being turned off inside their head. It is sometimes possible to switch on from the off state by taking an extra dose of treatment, but even this maybe ineffective. The Madopar Dispersible preparation is more helpful in this switching effect than the ordinary levodopa preparations because it produces a more rapid surge in the blood level of levodopa.

The swings from off to on can occur several times per day. At worst, they have no obvious relationship to the timing of the treatments but they often become more frequent as the day progresses. Yo-yo-ing is a very colourful term that has been used to describe this pattern of rapid sudden swing from mobility to immobility in the worst sufferers of the condition. The swings in the ability to move may be accompanied by changes in other symptoms; with the development of the off state, some people notice an increase in apathy and depression, difficulty in passing urine, visual disturbances and even pain in the limbs.

Treatment of the on/off syndrome is difficult. The first line measures are those described under end-of-dose deterioration detailed above; that is, increased frequency of dosage, entacapone, selegiline, dopamine agonists and slow release Madopar or Sinemet. Regrettably, the on/off syndrome is one of the major persisting causes of handicap in a proportion of people who have had Parkinson's disease for many years. Some success can be obtained with the drug apomorphine, which is given by injection (see below). Surgical treatments including brain transplants, pallidotomy and deep brain stimulation (described in the next chapter) have also been used for this complication of Parkinson's disease with variable success.

Dopamine agonists

Dopamine has been called a neurotransmitter because it is important for the transmission of messages from one nerve cell to another, rather like the transmission of electricity from one wire to another across a junction box. The dopamine is produced by one cell and is used to transmit messages to a second cell. The logic of dopamine treatment is to give back to the first cell the dopamine that is lacking. However, a second approach to treatment is to bypass the dopamine completely and to pass the message to the second cell, downstream, through the direct action of a different drug. These drugs, which act like dopamine, but bypass the dopamine-containing cell, have been called dopaminergic drugs or dopamine agonists.

The main dopamine agonists in current use are:

Bromocriptine (Parlodel)
Pergolide (Celance)
Ropinirole (Requip)
Cabergoline (Cabaser)
Pramipexole (Mirapexin)

Lysuride was used in the past but is no longer available in the United Kingdom. Apomorphine is a special dopamine agonist that is given by subcutaneous injection (see later in this chapter).

Although the dopamine agonists all act in a similar way, by

bypassing the dopamine-containing cell, they differ slightly in the way that they work. A single dose of some drugs, such as cabergoline, lasts for a longer time than other drugs, such as bromocriptine. Drugs which act for longer between doses can be particularly helpful in the treatment of response fluctuations, such as the on/off syndrome. The drug cabergoline is particularly beneficial in this respect because each dose of the drug seems to last for over twenty-four hours. These dopamine agonist drugs also differ somewhat in their side-effects. Although they can all produce similar side-effects, certain of these side-effects may be less common with one drug than another. For example, pergolide seems to produce fewer hallucinations than does lysuride. Obviously the makers of new drugs want to produce treatments that have the greatest beneficial effect with the fewest side-effects. This is one reason why new drugs, even of a similar type, are still appearing on the market. Amongst the dopamine agonists, my personal preference at the time of writing is for cabergoline.

Interestingly, the first study of the effects of a dopaminergic drug occurred before the development of levodopa therapy but it was really only in the 1970s that treatment with bromocriptine became established as a useful treatment for Parkinson's disease and the first of the dopamine agonist type of treatment. These drugs are now fully established as effective treatments alongside levodopa.

Recent research has raised some concerns about the possible long-term effects of levodopa treatment. It has been suggested that the use of levodopa, particularly in high doses, over many years may increase the risk of development of dyskinesias (see Chapter 5) later in the course of the condition. This is still not proven so you should not be alarmed if you are taking levodopa therapy (for example, Madopar or Sinemet), particularly since this treatment is generally more effective than other drugs available. However, the possibility that levodopa may, in some people, create problems in the long-term has led most doctors to use it in the lowest dose that is necessary. Furthermore, dopamine agonist drugs are now much more often used as first-line treatment in patients who can tolerate them and gain benefit from them. Some recent studies have shown that dyskinesias develop less frequently in patients who are taking only a dopamine agonist drug over the first five years of the condition,

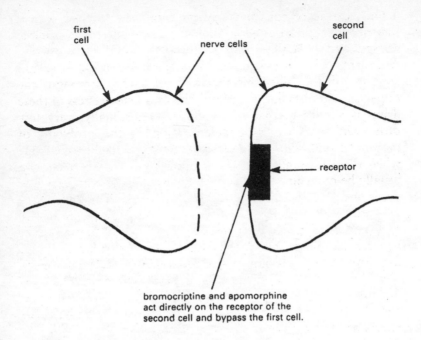

first
cell

nerve cells

second
cell

receptor

bromocriptine and apomorphine
act directly on the receptor of the
second cell and bypass the first cell.

Action of bromocriptine/apomorphine

when compared to people who are taking levodopa. What is not so clear is whether the dopamine agonist is truly preventing the development of dyskinesias by some protective effect on the brain or whether the drugs simply produce dyskinesias as a side effect less frequently than does levodopa. It may be that those people who are going to get dyskinesias on levodopa after say five years of Parkinson's would do so whether or not they had been taking only a dopamine agonist beforehand.

Another problem is that it is rarely possible to stay on a dopamine agonist as the only effective treatment for more than a few years and usually levodopa has to be added. Those people who are going to get dyskinesias will probably get them in any event when the levodopa therapy is added and previous treatment with dopamine agonists may make no different to this risk.

One reason for not using dopamine agonists on their own is that people seem to develop unpleasant side-effects – dizziness, nausea and generally feeling unwell – soon after starting treatment, even on low doses. As I have said, the nature and severity of the side-effects differs somewhat amongst the dopamine agonists but, in general, the list of side-effects of these drugs is similar to that of levodopa. Occasionally, very low doses can seem to cause deterioration in the problems of movement in Parkinson's disease but these are readily overcome when the doses increase. The more common side-effects can usually be overcome to a large degree by starting with very low doses and building up the dose gradually over a few weeks; if you have previously tried a dopamine agonist drug and were unable to take it because of the side-effects, you may find that you can get on to reasonable doses by building up the dose much more slowly. Some doctors routinely prescribe domperidone, which is an anti-sickness drug, when one of these drugs is first prescribed. Domperidone blocks the side effects of the drugs and is used routinely by these doctors to ensure that the side effects do not develop in the first place. Most people find that the side effects disappear after they have been taking the drugs for several weeks; under these circumstances, the domperidone can then be stopped. Other doctors only prescribe domperidone when the side effects develop. For people who are treated with reasonable doses of a dopamine agonist alone, they experience improvement in most of the features of Parkinson's disease, in a similar way to treatment with levodopa. The improvement covers the symptoms of akinesia, rigidity and sometimes tremor, but has least effect against poor balance and gait. Some research is investigating the possibility that drugs such as pergolide may slow down the progression of Parkinson's disease and avoid some of the later complications, such as dyskinesia and on/off swings.

Dopamine agonists are also used in combination with levodopa and have particular value in the following circumstances:

• Firstly, they can allow you to reduce the total daily dose of levodopa; this can be helpful for some patients who seem to need large doses of levodopa in order to get about, but who develop intolerable side-effects. The combination of levodopa and a dopamine agonist seems to provide as much help to their mobility, without provoking as many side-effects, as do large doses of levodopa alone.

- The drugs can be helpful for treatment of on/off fluctuations. The dopamine agonists generally have a longer duration of action than does levodopa, so can smooth out the switches from on to off that often occur in people treated with levodopa alone. This is particularly so when the swings appear to have a clear relationship to the timing of treatment, such as in end-of-dose deterioration. However, even in more chaotic on/off swings, the addition of a dopamine agonist can smooth things out over the course of the day.
- Dopamine agonist drugs can help with some of the problems that occur at night or in the early morning; for example, people who have difficulty in turning over in bed may gain relief from a night-time dose of cabergoline because the drug continues to act during the night. Similarly, early morning dystonia (see Chapter 5) can be dramatically helped by a night-time dose of cabergoline.
- Dopamine agonists may also help the dystonia associated with the disease and can help some of the pains that occur during the off periods.

The side-effects of dopamine agonists are very similar to those of levodopa. In the short term the side-effects tend to be more common with higher doses; these include nausea, vomiting, fall in blood pressure on standing, confusion, hallucination, sedation and general feelings of being unwell. Sometimes blurred vision, a dry mouth, leg cramps, skin flushes and rashes may develop. The side-effects of nausea and vomiting can be helped by treatment with domperidone (Motilium), whilst many of the other side effects are only prominent soon after beginning treatment, and settle as the drug is continued.

High doses of the drug may produce dyskinesias, in the same way as levodopa (see above). However, as discussed above, dyskinesias seem to be less common in patients who are able to tolerate a dopamine agonist as the only effective treatment. Many doctors begin treatment with a dopamine agonist, particularly in younger patients, but virtually all such patients ultimately end up on levodopa as well.

Selegiline

Selegiline is a drug that has very little effect in relieving the symptoms of Parkinson's disease when taken on its own. Its main use is as an addition to treatment with levodopa, particularly for people who experience fluctuations in their mobility through the day (see page 71). Normally, the body will break down and dispose of dopamine after it has been produced. One of the chemicals (known as enzymes) which causes this breakdown of dopamine is called monoamine oxidase. The drug selegiline interferes with this process so that the amount of dopamine available for transmitting messages in the brain is increased. Each dose of levodopa also acts for a longer period of time because of selegiline's interference with the body's breakdown mechanisms. The drug is particularly useful for the treatment of end-of-dose deterioration, and has some benefit in the treatment of problems associated with sleep and the early morning, such as difficulty in turning in bed and early morning dystonia. It may be of some help to people with on/off swings but the more severe forms of this condition are, unfortunately, helped little by selegiline.

Selegiline is prescribed in 5-mg tablets; unlike most other treatments for Parkinson's disease, there is not much variation in dosage. Two 5-mg tablets daily are all that is required. The drug has relatively few side-effects, but these include dry mouth, light-headedness, sleeplessness and nausea. But as the drug increases the body levels of dopamine it can thus provoke side-effects due directly to levodopa.

Selegiline has undergone renewed interest because of a possible effect on slowing down the rate of progression of Parkinson's disease. The substance MPTP has been found to be poisonous to the parts of the brain that are abnormal in Parkinson's disease, so that this poison can produce a condition very similar to that of Parkinson's disease (see Chapters 2 and 4). It has been found that the drug selegiline will interfere with the actions of MPTP on the cells of the basal ganglia. Although Parkinson's disease is not caused by MPTP, observations from the effects of MPTP poisoning suggested to researchers that another, similar poison may be present in the environment, or may accumulate within the body, and may cause Parkinson's disease. If so, then maybe selegiline would prevent accumulation of this poison within the brain and may prevent the development of Parkinson's disease. Dopamine is also broken down by cells in the brain after it has been released and the products of this breakdown may be toxic to dopamine-containing cells in the brain. Breakdown of dopamine by these mechanisms is also blocked by selegiline so that, in theory, selegiline could have a protective effect on the brain cells through this mechanism as well.

It is important to realise that a protective effect of selegiline on the brain is completely unproven. However, studies have been carried out in the United States to find out if selegiline will slow down the rate of progression of the disease. Selegiline 10 mg daily was given to untreated patients early in the course of the disease and compared with the effects of a placebo, or dummy tablet. Doctors kept observing the patients until they needed treatment with levodopa and found that the use of selegiline meant that it was almost twice as long before levodopa became necessary. Because selegiline on its own has very little effect on most of the symptoms of Parkinson's disease, this research has suggested that the drug may slow down the rate at which the changes of Parkinson's disease in the brain get worse. But there is another interpretation – the drug could make people feel better in a way that has not yet been fully recognized and this beneficial feeling could delay the need for levodopa treatment without affecting the process of the disease itself. If so, the drug is just acting as another treatment for symptoms without getting at the real cause of the disease.

Some doctors feel that selegiline should be given when the disease is diagnosed. However, at the time of writing, the effect of the drug on the brain changes of Parkinson's disease is still something of an open question and we cannot be sure of any long-term disadvantages. In fact, another study in the United Kingdom suggested that selegiline has no protective effects but, by contrast, may have a deleterious effect in the long term (see page 62). It is important that research continues into this important question before selegiline can be considered in any way a 'cure' or even a factor that will definitely prevent further deterioration from the disease in all patients with Parkinson's disease. More recent studies from the USA suggest that any protective effect is operative only in the first few years of the condition.

COMT inhibitors

COMT (which stands for Catechol-O-Methyl-Transferase) is an enzyme in the blood and the brain which causes breakdown of levodopa and dopamine. In this respect it is similar to monoamine oxidase, an enzyme which is blocked by selegiline (see above) although it works by a different mechanism. A drug which blocked the action of COMT would increase the availability of the drug levodopa for conversion into the active brain chemical dopamine, and would also increase the brain levels of dopamine by preventing its breakdown. Two drugs have been developed which work through this route: tolcapone and entacapone. Tolcapone was marketed for a while but was withdrawn when it was found to damage the liver in a few patients. The only drug now available is entacapone.

Entacapone is useful because it reduces the amount of levodopa that has to be given to achieve the same brain levels of dopamine. Moreover, it helps some of the response fluctuations, such as end of dose deterioration, because it prolongs the action of each levodopa dose by preventing the breakdown of levodopa and dopamine. Side effects are similar to those of levodopa but it may also produce diarrhoea. It also discolours the urine.

Apomorphine

Apomorphine is, in fact, a dopamine agonist drug (see page 72), but has been included in a separate category in this book because it is used and given in quite a different way from the other dopamine agonists that have been described.

- Apomorphine is never used except in the more advanced cases of Parkinson's disease.
- The drug has to be given by an injection of liquid under the skin because it cannot be taken in tablet form, although a tablet that dissolves under the tongue and preparations of the drug that can be taken through some other route, such as a nasal spray or skin patch, may soon become available.

Neurologists use apomorphine for the treatment of severe on/off swings when there seems to be little benefit from any other treatment.

The drug can be injected under the skin by one of two methods. The Penject method uses a syringe that can be adjusted so that a standard dose is given whenever a button at one end is pressed. When the syringe is filled with the drug it contains sufficient to provide several individual doses. The Penject is so-called because it is about the size of a large ballpoint pen and can be stored in the pocket, secured by a clip. The syringe is usually kept by a relative, who provides an injection to the Parkinsonian sufferer whenever he switches from an on to an off phase.

The second method involves the use of a pump system. The modern pumps are small, about the size of the smallest mobile phones. The pump is filled with the drug in liquid form, similarly to the Penject. The pump unit is then carried by the patient, strapped around the waist. Leading from the pump is a tube which passes directly to a needle placed under the skin and secured by sticking plaster. The pump is operated by a small battery and delivers the drug at a set rate continuously through the day. This method is more suitable for people who have very frequent on/off swings.

With both of these methods, relatives have to be taught how to fill and clean the syringe and how to perform the subcutaneous injection. However, almost everyone learns these procedures very quickly, and you should not be alarmed at the prospect if your doctor suggests it. If there are problems a district nurse may be available to put the needle in each morning. The injection carries no more pain than a needle prick, while the carrying of the pump with its attached needle is entirely painless. So you should not be alarmed at the thought of inflicting pain on a close relative if you are required to carry out these injections. The method of injection under the skin is essentially the same as that used by diabetic patients who inject insulin – although the drug is, of course, quite different.

Use of apomorphine can considerably help patients who have severe on/off swings. Side effects of the drugs are similar to those of levodopa and the dopamine agonists (see pages 68–70 and 74). Domperidone, a drug to prevent vomiting, is always taken with apomorphine treatment because, without it, the apomorphine can produce unpleasant nausea and vomiting. Domperidone is, however, very effective at preventing these side-effects.

Recently, much smaller doses of apomorphine have been found to help erectile impotence in men.

Other drug treatments

- Baclofen is a drug more commonly used in diseases other than Parkinson's disease, in order to relieve muscle spasm. The drug may, however, be helpful to patients with Parkinson's disease who suffer from painful dystonias or nocturnal cramps.

- Antidepressant drugs – many patients with Parkinson's disease develop depression, not only because of the effects of Parkinson's disease on their life but also because of chemical changes within the brain (see Chapter 6). Sometimes it is necessary to treat the depression separately from the difficulties in movement, and a variety of antidepressant drugs is available for this purpose. The presence of depression should always be considered in patients with Parkinson's disease. You should raise the question with your doctor if you have any concern about the possibility of depression in yourself or your relatives. Antidepressant treatment can also be helpful in relieving some of the sensory symptoms of Parkinson's disease, such as burning, itching, pricking, tingling and pins and needles.

- Painkillers and anti-arthritic drugs – pain and stiffness are prominent features of uncomplicated Parkinson's disease. However, the lack of mobility, altered posture and general muscle stiffness produced by this disease may also worsen pain arising from underlying wear and tear on the joints that is so common with increasing age, with or without the burden of additional Parkinson's disease. Many different drugs exist for the treatment of this sort of joint pain, so you should raise the question with your doctor if you are having particular problems with pain and stiffness that do not seem to be helped by your treatment for Parkinson's disease.

- Although tranquillisers and sleeping tablets are occasionally helpful for the treatment of some of the stiffness, tingling and burning and for the disturbed sleep that results from Parkinson's disease, they are best avoided, if possible. There are often other methods of dealing with these problems, and these drugs can become addictive in the long term. Small doses of the anti-depressant drug, amitriptyline may help insomnia in Parkinson's disease.

- When confusion and hallucinations occur, either as part of Parkinson's disease or its treatment, it is sometimes necessary to treat these symptoms with a different type of drug, sometimes called neuroleptics. The drugs include chlorpromazine, haloperidol, sulpiride risperidone, quetiapine, olanzapine and clozapine. Most of these drugs work by blocking the effects of dopamine in the brain so they can easily make the problems with movement worse, even though they help these other features. These drugs differ in the extent to which they will cause movement problems but the vast majority of them do, often to a great extent. Doctors use these drugs for the treatment of confusion and hallucinations only in very small doses. You should only take these drugs under medical supervision and never be tempted to change the dose without the approval of your doctor.

The neuroleptics which cause the fewest problems with movement and hence are best in dealing with hallucinations, are quetiapine, clozapine and olanzopine. However, patients taking clozapine require close supervision and regular blood tests because it can effect the white cells in the blood.

Donepezil, galantamine and rivastigmine are drugs that have been licensed for treatment of the memory loss of Alzheimer's disease. They provide some help but do not completely correct the problem. Experience of these drugs in the memory problems of Parkinson's disease is limited but there is some evidence that they have a similar beneficial effect. They may also suppress the hallucinations.

The problem of fall in blood pressure on standing, causing dizziness, (see Chapter 7) can be helped by drugs that increase the blood pressure. These drugs include ephedrine and fludrocortisone. It is important that a doctor carefully monitors their use because they can have deleterious effects on the heart and circulation.

9

Other treatments

In the previous chapter we discussed the various medicines that are available for the treatment of Parkinson's disease. However, medication is not the only way in which help can be offered to suffererers. Other treatments include surgical operations, diet, and a broad category of treatments that we loosely call rehabilitation. Rehabilitation not only includes physiotherapy, occupational therapy, speech therapy and social support; it also includes an important area, often forgotten – the giving of advice, the discussion of problems and the provision of information.

Operations for Parkinson's disease

When people think of a surgical operation they usually think of something that provides an instant 'cure', such as removal of the appendix for appendicitis. It is not surprising, therefore, that people tend to be keener to seek some sort of operation for their disease than accepting the prospects of taking tablets every day for the rest of their lives. For Parkinson's disease, however, the situation is not that simple. Now that levodopa and the other effective drugs have been discovered, the most effective treatment for the vast majority of patients is taking regular medication.

Sometimes, though, the symptoms of Parkinson's disease can be helped by surgery. There are now two main types of operation that are used – stereotactic surgery and the more recent operation of brain transplants, described below.

Stereotactic surgery

Brain operations for Parkinson's disease began just before the Second World War and were very popular during the 1940s and 1950s, prior to the discovery of levodopa in the 1960s.

Although the risk of stroke in Parkinson's disease is no greater than in anyone else, the first clue to successful surgery was given by the unfortunate coincidence of a stroke in people who also suffered from Parkinson's disease. When the stroke damaged a small area of the basal ganglia, the tremor of Parkinson's disease tended to disappear. This accident of nature prompted surgeons to try the effect on the symptoms of Parkinson's disease of deliberate damage to these brain regions. The operations were found to reduce the tremor and rigidity quite markedly, although they did not affect the akinesia. As the operations became more refined, surgeons learnt precisely where to create the damage in order to produce the best effects. Ultimately they were able to achieve dramatic improvements with only very small areas of damage.

The operation is carried out by placing a fine needle into the basal ganglia and passing something like an electric current through it. This produces a very localized area of heat, which damages the nerve cells around it. Surgeons know exactly where to produce this damage by using equipment very much like a map and a compass; using X-ray techniques, they build up a map of the patient's brain and the 'compass' shows them in which direction, and for how far, they should pass their needle. The term stereotactic refers to this use of a 'map' and 'compass'.

There are several types of stereotactic operation which are given names according to the region of the brain that is deliberately damaged by the operation. The commonest stereotactic operation, until recently, is known as thalamotomy. Thalamotomy is able to abolish tremor and rigidity in virtually four-fifths of the people who undergo operations. However, most operations are done on only one side of the brain, so the relief affects only one side of the body. The operation is therefore particularly useful for people who have signs of Parkinson's disease confined to one side of the body. The operation can produce relief of the tremor for many years, but it does not prevent tremor or rigidity developing on the other side of the body. In addition, the operation has no effect on akinesia, which is probably the most disabling aspect of Parkinson's disease.

With the development of levodopa the operation has become much less popular; three-quarters of the hospital departments that used to carry out these operations have now ceased to do so. The operation is still available, however, for certain selected people who have problems that cannot be eased in any other way. In brief, the operation is nowadays occasionally considered for the following people:

- Those with severe tremor or rigidity but relatively little akinesia or gait disturbance.
- Those whose symptoms affect only one side of the body.
- Those who show no improvement with levodopa or other anti-Parkinsonian drugs.
- Those who develop very troublesome side-effects.
- Younger rather than older people.
- Those with severe dyskinesia secondary to levodopa.

Thalamotomy can improve levodopa dyskinesias but it does not affect end-of-dose deterioration or the on/off phenomenon (see Chapter 8). More recently a new stereotactic operation, known as pallidotomy, has become popular. The small area of damage made in the brain is different from that in thalamotomy and the effects on Parkinson's disability appear to be better. Pallidotomy seems to improve particularly the akinesia and rigidity, rather than the tremor. Since it is the akinesia and rigidity that are the more disabling aspects of Parkinson's disease for most sufferers, pallidotomy has the promise of being a better operation for most patients. In addition, the operation seems to reduce substantially the dyskinesias and on/off swings that constitute so much of the disability in chronic Parkinson's disease. Although the operation was first done many years ago, it has only fairly recently undergone a revival and its effects are still under investigation. However, at the time of writing, this operation is being carried out in many centres in the United Kingdom, Europe and the United States and the results do seem to be promising. One thing that we do not know, however, is how long the benefit will last and whether there are any long-term side-effects from the operation. At the moment the operation is being reserved for patients who have severe Parkinson's disease that is not helped by any other form of treatment, but it may well be that it becomes more available to other patients if its initial promises are fulfilled after a few more years' observation.

It should be remembered that stereotactic surgery is an operation on the brain and is always a potentially dangerous procedure; fortunately, complications are rare, but occasionally they can be serious. As well as the general risks of an operation on the head, stereotactic surgery has some special unwanted after-effects, some more serious than others; these include tiredness, poor memory and concentration, twitching movements of the arm and leg, slurring of speech and epilepsy. Usually these problems last only a few days or weeks and are followed by complete recovery; rarely, however, they are longer lasting.

Another type of surgical treatment that has recently been introduced and is still undergoing investigation is similar to the procedures just described in that an electrode is placed deep into parts of the brain that are known to be functioning wrongly in Parkinson's disease. However, in this type of operation, known as deep brain stimulation the particular brain region is not destroyed by an electric current. Instead, a lower strength current is applied which stimulates the brain area but does not destroy it. The electrical stimulation is maintained constantly through a sort of battery attached to the electrode outside the body. By adjusting the strength of the electrical current it is possible to stop the functioning of that region of the brain without actually destroying it. The effects of this sort of operation are similar to the more conventional types of surgery where a permanent area of brain damage is produced, but the advantage is that the electric current can be turned off if, for example, side-effects develop or the condition of the patient changes so that the treatment is no longer suitable. Under these circumstances the electrode can be removed with no permanent effects on the brain and a different form of treatment, which may include chronic stimulation of another brain region, can be introduced instead. In addition, unlike the types of operation that lead to permanent damage, the strength of the electric current can be adjusted to block the function of the particular brain region to just the right amount to suit the symptoms of an individual patient. Again, this type of operation is relatively new, and is still undergoing evaluation to establish the long-term benefits and disadvantages.

It should be remembered that stereotactic surgery became less popular because drugs have taken its place as a more effective and safer treatment. Only a very small minority of people with Parkinson's disease are now more likely to benefit from this sort of operation than from some adjustment of their drug treatment

– it is always worth a very enthusiastic attempt to get the drug treatment right before embarking on surgery.

Brain transplants

In the late 1970s scientists began to explore ways in which the area of brain damaged in Parkinson's disease could be repaired, so that people would not have to take drugs for the rest of their life. This became a particularly important issue when they began to see some of the unexpected problems associated with years of drug treatment. They then showed in rats that damage to the dopamine cells of the basal ganglia could be partially repaired by transplanting dopamine cells from other parts of the body. These cells were obtained from two places – the adrenal gland, which sits just above the kidney, and the substantia nigra (the area damaged in Parkinson's disease) from dead, unborn foetuses. Since then, scientists have shown that similar transplants can improve the symptoms of Parkinsonism produced by MPTP in animals (Chapter 4). As expected, the improvement seems to occur because the transplant increases the dopamine levels in the brain.

Between 1982 and 1985 four patients in Sweden were given grafts of the adrenal gland in an attempt to improve their severe Parkinson's disease. These patients all improved, but the effects were not long-lasting – several months after the operation they had all reverted to their previous Parkinsonian state. More recently, surgeons in Mexico claimed a much greater success using a similar operation. Surgeons in various places throughout the world, including the United States and the United Kingdom, have since performed a number of similar operations and doctors are now waiting to see for how long people improve, if at all. At the time of writing it appears that some people do improve after surgery, but the hopes from the early operations may not be quite fulfilled. Special techniques show that the grafts will survive and grow in the Parkinsonian brain, but not all grafts do so, and many simply fail to produce dopamine. (Strangely enough, patients sometimes improve even though these techniques show no production of dopamine, so the operations may be working in a way quite different from that which was imagined when the graft was devised in the first place.)

It has certainly been the experience to date that most patients need to continue their anti-Parkinsonian drugs after the operation, even if at a reduced dosage. In addition, some patients fail to show any benefit whatever, and some suffer side-effects from the surgery and are made worse as a result. Even for those people who do show definite benefit it is not clear for how long this improvement continues after surgery; despite initial improvement some patients have been seen to deteriorate over the 12 months after surgery, so that they are back to their preoperative state by one year after operation.

Do remember that the benefits from any operation have to be weighed against the side-effects, and 'brain transplants' are an even more major surgical procedure than the stereotactic operations described earlier in this chapter. Everyone looks for the miracle cure, but it is important to weigh up the effects of any treatment with a careful assessment of the benefits and risks. At the moment you would be wise to discuss the pros and cons very carefully with your doctor before rushing in to have this sort of operation carried out on yourself.

Some further points about 'brain transplants' should also be clarified. Firstly, the term 'brain transplant' is really incorrect. It is not, of course, the whole brain that is transplanted, only a small piece of nervous tissue that is grafted into the brain of the patient. The more accurate term is neural graft. Secondly, these operations are very carefully supervised, for ethical reasons. Some operations are carried out using the substantia nigra from human foetuses, and the ethics of this situation are obviously very personal. All such surgical procedures must be approved by an ethical committee, present in every city and consisting of medical and non-medical people. This does not mean, of course, that you have to agree with these committees, and everyone should make their own personal decision; however, these panels review any new venture very carefully, to the best of their ability, so the ethical question concerning neural grafting has certainly been reviewed from a number of different angles by people of differing attitudes. In addition, the foetuses are obtained from abortions that have been carried out for reasons quite separate from the neural grafting for Parkinson's disease; consent to the use of the foetuses is always obtained, and the brain transplant procedure does not influence in any way the reasons for carrying out the abortion in the first place.

At the time of writing, researchers are still working on better ways to improve Parkinson's disease by the neural graft technique. Firstly, they are trying to find ways to prevent the graft from dying, which usually happens because the brain recognizes the implanted graft as 'foreign' and rejects it. This form of research is centred around methods to prevent the graft rejection, similar to treatments that have been used to prevent rejection of kidney grafts. Secondly, researchers are trying to develop grafts that do not depend upon the use of aborted foetuses. Apart from the ethical question, one neural graft to a single patient requires the use of several foetuses which is not a practical proposition if the treatment were to become widespread. Thus, scientists are trying to develop ways to grow dopamine cells outside the body in the laboratory. These would then act as a source of material for neural grafting and would not involve the use of aborted foetuses. Stem cells are cells that have the potential to develop into lots of different kinds of cells in the brain, including dopamine-producing cells. Researchers are currently testing the benefit of implanting stem cells into the brain of Parkinson's sufferers.

What about the future?

Parkinson's disease is a very active research area and the prospects for more effective treatments over the years to come are good. Firstly, all of our bodily processes are controlled by our genetic make-up. Although, in most cases of Parkinson's disease, we cannot identify a single gene abnormality that causes the condition, it may nevertheless be possible to modify in some way those genes that control the production of dopamine. If we could get at the genes in the dopamine, then it would open a new avenue for treatment of this condition. Research is being carried out into this possibility at the time of writing. Secondly, we have always thought that the brain, once damaged, is incapable of repairing itself. In contrast to other areas of the body (such as the skin) which can 'heal up' when damaged, this does not seem to happen in the nervous system. However, recently scientists have discovered that it may be possible to persuade the brain to repair itself under some conditions. This research is still in its early stages but it does lend hope to the prospect that treatment in the future may be geared towards an actual repair of the cells that are damaged in Parkinson's disease. Thirdly, research using selegiline has stimulated our efforts to find drugs that will restrict ongoing damage to the cells of the substantia nigra. The idea of this sort of treatment is to prevent progression of the disease once it has been diagnosed, and to avoid many of the later complications that form much of the disability in chronic Parkinson's disease and which may be resistant to available treatments. Unlike currently available drug treatments, which simply replace the chemicals that are lost from the damaged cells, these new sorts of treatment are targeted at the heart of the problem, and theoretically could avoid the need for the sorts of drugs that we use now. Although this research is going on, it is important to realise that an active treatment is still quite a long way off. Drugs are still the most effective treatments, and possibly the operations discussed earlier.

Can diet affect Parkinson's disease?

If you have Parkinson's disease, you should maintain your general health by eating a healthy balanced diet. This is good advice for everyone, whether or not they have the disease, but if you do have it you should be particularly keen to keep your body in good general trim.

If you have difficulty in swallowing you should be sure to eat an adequate diet in some other form. One simple way is to mince up the food or to purée it in a liquidizer. If you have severe swallowing problems, then you can obtain wholefood compounds in liquid form that give you most of your necessary nutrition, including vitamins and minerals, for the whole day. These can be obtained from your local chemist, or your doctor will advise you.

If you do have swallowing problems be sure that they do not make you miss your medication. The dispersible form of Madopar can be suspended in water and is often helpful for people who are unable to swallow capsules or tablets. There is no harm in taking regular vitamin supplements, such as many people do whether or not they have Parkinson's disease; however you should be careful not to take large doses of vitamin B6 (pyridoxine) because this can interfere with the action of levodopa and thus upset your drug treatment.

One sort of problem may be particularly helped by a change

of diet. It has been found that people who have marked on/off swings can be improved if they reduce the quantity of protein in their diet. Protein is particularly concentrated in meat, fish, milk and some vegetables; if you have marked on/off swings eliminating these items from your diet may increase the 'on' times, and make the swings from 'on' to 'off' less dramatic. This change of diet can be combined with a change of tablets. But you must realise that, although a low-protein diet may be helpful for the on/off swings, it is not likely to help people with Parkinson's disease who do not have this particular problem. Your doctor will be able to provide you with a diet sheet to highlight foods that have a high protein content, or he can refer you to a dietician within your area who can advise you further.

Be a little aware of new 'miracle cures' which are advertised from time to time and often involve some form of dietary supplement. All of us, doctors included, should keep an open mind about any treatment which is potentially helpful for Parkinson's disease. However, many of us have seen these 'miracle cures' come and later go, after they had been proved ineffective. Sometimes treatments are promoted prematurely from misplaced enthusiasm and probably as in all aspects of life sometimes from frank deception in order to make money. There is no harm in taking treatment which is safe and cheap provided you keep an open mind and do not allow yourself to generate high and possibly false hopes. All treatments need to be carefully evaluated before we can be confident of their effectiveness, which is why doctors seem sceptical at unorthodox treatments that have not been proven.

Help with physical disability

Under this heading we will look at physiotherapy, occupational therapy and speech therapy. All will usually be available at your local district general hospital, and sometimes at your health centre.

Often such treatment is carried out on a one-to-one basis, with a therapist; occasionally, though, special support groups are organized for people with Parkinson's disease. If you are fortunate enough to have access to such a group, you may find it very helpful, as you can share your problems with others who have similar difficulties and discuss various solutions.

Physiotherapy

Physiotherapy means treatment using physical means; for example, these techniques involve exercise, manipulation and the application of heat or other forms of stimulation to inflamed areas. In Parkinson's disease physiotherapy can be useful in the following ways:

- To maintain loose joints and muscles.
- To improve co-ordination and dexterity of the hands.
- To improve posture and increase awareness of body position.
- To improve control of breathing.
- To teach techniques to improve walking.
- To teach easier, more efficient ways of coping with activities of daily life.
- To offer general advice and support.

It is probably a good idea for the patient with Parkinson's disease to take regular exercise. Specially taught exercises are best because these provide the maximum benefit in the shortest time. Ideally, every patient with Parkinson's disease should see a physiotherapist to learn these exercises but, regrettably, this is not always possible. Exercise sheets are, however, available from your doctor, physiotherapist or local branch of the Parkinson's Disease Society. Regular exercise will help to reduce the risk of chest infections, will help constipation and will improve cramps and poor circulation in the legs.

Occupational therapy

Occupational therapy is very much linked to physical therapy, but stresses more the way in which we can adapt ourselves to everyday life, within the limits of our disability. Occupational therapy can show you how to plan your home to make daily tasks more acceptable in three ways – by making it safer, easier and more enjoyable.

Physical therapy and occupational therapy can provide you with physical aids to help you in your day-to-day life; for example, people who have difficulty in manipulating a knife and fork can be helped considerably if they are given implements with larger handles that they can grip more easily. For people who have difficulty in walking, walking sticks or walking frames can be provided (interestingly, for the patient with Parkinson's disease, these are not always helpful – if they are not used quite precisely they get in the way and increase rather than decrease the problems with balance).

Sometimes the severely disabled person must accept the use of a wheelchair. Many people are reluctant to do this because they see it as a sign of loss of independence. Nevertheless, if you or your relative is severely disabled you should consider the use of a wheelchair, because this will allow you to get out of the house much more, and increase rather than decrease your freedom.

Speech therapy

Speech therapy is available for people who have slurring of speech or difficulty in expression. The treatment can provide training in control of the voice so that words do not run into each other, can help increase the speech volume and bring about an improvement in confidence. Speech therapists are also skilled in the provision of communication aids. For the unfortunate few whose speech disturbance is so bad that they cannot make themselves understood orally, machines are available that will assist in communication; for example, portable microphones and amplifiers can be worn about the neck or attached to clothing to help the particular problem of low speech volume. In other cases, small typewriters can be used to bypass speech altogether. These have been specially adapted so that they can be used by someone with poor control of the limbs, and there are often visual displays so that the message can be easily read.

Help with emotional and psychological problems

You would be a lucky person if you did not have some emotional or psychological reaction to the news that you, or a close relative, had Parkinson's disease. You would also be fortunate if you did not develop some additional reaction over the following years. Having Parkinson's disease inevitably alters one's life, whether in minor or major form, so the vast majority of people do develop some reaction. Regrettably, this aspect of the illness is often overlooked, despite the fact that the reactions often affect both the person with Parkinson's disease and their family.

The news of the diagnosis itself is often a shock. None of us wishes to become ill or to learn that we have a condition that may get worse, and for which we will need to take regular tablets. Some people express resentment under these circumstances; they may find it difficult to accept the diagnosis, and do their best to prove their doctor wrong. Of course, sometimes doctors are wrong, and if you have real doubts you would be wise to seek a second opinion. But some people relentlessly seek third, fourth or fifth opinions, in the belief that they can get rid of the diagnosis. However, once the diagnosis is certain, it is better to come to terms with it rather than to fight it.

Sometimes the news provokes feelings of anger. Many people are around retirement age when they develop Parkinson's disease and, after a lifetime of hard work, they see the condition as interfering with their retirement plans. In contrast, young people may see themselves thwarted in their ambitions for themselves and their family at the prime of their lives. These are obviously understandable reactions, but again not helpful in the long term. Some people have an opposite reaction, with feelings of worthlessness – that they can no longer contribute to their family, friends or work.

The best way to deal with these feelings is by information; most people are best able to come to terms with their altered situation if they are given the necessary facts. It is lack of knowledge about a condition, its treatment and the future prospects that leads to anxiety because the afflicted person does not have the necessary information on which to base their judgment.

A new set of reactions can occur in response to physical limitations. The physical difficulties, which particularly affect people later in the disease, can affect both the patients and their families. Many people become depressed because they are no longer able to carry out a task that they could previously do quite easily (see Chapter 6). As physical limitations develop, you may find that you have to give up hobbies, social activities or even your job. The resulting depression will itself, in turn, produce loss of drive, energy and initiative, which will add to your inability to cope with everyday life. A vicious circle soon develops in which the physical disability leads to depression and the depression leads to fatigue and apathy, which further reduces your ability to cope.

You may have been the leader of the family, but now you have to take a more dependent role. Your family may have been used to your taking control, but now find they have to make many of the decisions and carry out the household tasks themselves. Some relatives of patients with Parkinson's disease are shocked to find that they have to fit electric plugs, change light bulbs or do the mending for the first time in their lives. These changes can produce strain in even the most stable families. Sometimes, patients feel as if they are being judged by their family; or they may feel guilty. A close family member of the patient may resent his or her physical disability; they may choose to ignore the problem, become impatient or even sometimes abusive. These reactions can affect not only the husband or wife but also the children of the affected person, particularly if the children are grown up and independent but are required to contribute their efforts (or their money) to the problems of the Parkinsonian sufferer.

It is not possible to provide a simple formula to deal with these problems. However, it is essential to recognize that they do occur, even in the best families. The problems should be discussed freely amongst all members of the family, including the patients themselves. The problems of everyday life can sometimes be helped by setting a timetable for each person so that the difficulties become incorporated into a daily routine. You should aim for the best quality of life. Do not try to be too ambitious but be content with small achievements. If you are the patient, accept help in so far as you need it but try not to become dependent on others for everything you do – try to keep something for yourself, however small this may be.

Help with social problems

When someone becomes physically disabled from Parkinson's disease or severe emotional reactions develop within themselves or their family, everyday life is affected. But many such problems can be helped by simple attention to the living accommodation. For example:

- The household furniture can be modified to produce a safer environment.
- Objects can be moved a reasonable distance from commonly trodden routes.
- Polished floors or loose rugs, which may provoke falling, can be altered to safer floor coverings.
- Higher chairs will make it easier for a person with Parkinson's disease to stand up without assistance.
- Similarly, raising the seat may make them independent when going to the toilet.
- Handrails can be fitted on stairs, or wherever else appears necessary, to provide support.
- Cooker guards can be fitted to avoid accidental burning or scalding during cooking.
- Lighting should be bright, to minimize the risk of stumbling over unseen objects.
- Think about your pets – on the one hand they can be a great comfort if you are alone for long periods, but on the other hand a small dog or cat may get under your feet and cause you to fall.

Fortunately, very many people with Parkinson's disease do not have these physical limitations – they are completely independent. But others are dependent upon some sort of assistance in everyday life. Where a husband or wife is fit and able there is often less of a problem (but not always). Alternatively a grown-up son or daughter may be willing to provide support, either by frequent visits to the home or by having the Parkinson's sufferer in their own home.

Not all people are able to live together harmoniously, however, even though they may be related. You should therefore feel no sense of guilt if your personalities are different and the sharing of a home does not seem possible. The local authority is often able to provide warden-controlled flats or bungalows if the person is semi-independent, while other people can be looked after in residential nursing homes funded from the National Health Service or from private funds. As with all facilities, some nursing homes are very good and some are very bad, so you should visit the home in advance and obtain a clear picture of what is on offer. Advice on all these aspects of day-to-day life can be obtained from your local social worker. Your doctor, or the appropriate department of the local authority, will be able to help you to obtain this advice.

For the less serious problems it can be a great help to join a local support group, if there is one in your area. The Parkinson's Disease Society has a number of branches organized by local volunteers, usually patients and their relatives. Many of the simple day-to-day problems can be helped by talking to someone in a similar situation or by listening to a talk from an expert.

What about alternative medicines?

Acupuncture is a treatment that originated in China. It involves placing short sharp needles in the skin of key areas of the body. Acupuncture can help to relieve pain, so you may gain some benefit from this treatment if pain is a prominent feature of your condition. Such relief of pain can in turn help you to get about more easily, but the treatment is not likely to help you if you do not have pain.

Hypnosis can help to produce relaxation. We know that stress and mental agitation can make the symptoms of Parkinson's disease worse (although they do not cause the disease), so hypnosis may help if you are a particularly stressful or highly strung sort of person. For most people with Parkinson's disease, however, acupuncture and hypnosis are only of limited help. Yoga can help produce an attitude of relaxation, and it can also help because it is a form of exercise.

Homoeopathy is not a traditional treatment for Parkinson's disease, and most doctors do not have much experience of it.

Many of these alternative medicines may be helpful, but only as an addition to your drug treatment. Acupuncture, hypnosis and yoga can help in the manner described, but they will not affect some important features of Parkinson's disease, such as the akinesia. You should also be careful about accepting great claims for a new treatment of Parkinson's disease. We are all looking for the miracle cure, but some people get over-enthusiastic in their claims for new treatments and, regrettably, some people are willing to take advantage of the needs of others. Many false claims have been made about treatment in medicine, some of them just foolhardy but some of them deliberate.

Always speak to your doctor if you have heard of some new treatment that you think could be helpful.

What are drug holidays?

Occasionally some people do better with their treatment if they stop it all completely for a week or two and then start it again. This break from treatment, which has been called a drug holiday, can be a dangerous procedure, though. Obviously your symptoms of Parkinson's disease will get much worse when you stop your drugs – you may be unable to move at all, and could be at considerable risk. For this reason, drug holidays are only carried out in hospital and under close medical supervision. They are helpful for only a small proportion of people with Parkinson's disease, and most doctors in this country do not use this treatment at all routinely. Under no circumstances whatsoever must you stop your drugs of your own accord.

10

The most common questions

Most people have questions about their illness. Many doctors try to anticipate these questions by providing information without being asked. However, there is usually insufficient time at your doctor's appointment to cover all aspects of Parkinson's disease. Moreover, he or she would have to be a genius to anticipate all the questions a patient could possibly ask.

You may feel embarrassed or unwilling to ask your doctor for information, so, to help you, we have listed below the most common questions that are asked of the Medical Advisory Panel of the Parkinson's Disease Society. Sometimes a simple answer has been given. In many cases, however, we have also referred you to the part of the book that discusses this question more fully. If you do not find the answer in this book, please do not hesitate to ask your doctor, because you may find that the problem can be easily solved. It may even not have anything whatsoever to do with Parkinson's disease.

Causes

• *Can Parkinson's disease be caused by an injury to the head several years earlier?*
Head injury is very unlikely to be responsible for true Parkinson's disease, but it may cause a condition that resembles it – see Chapter 4.

• *Is Parkinson's disease hereditary?*
Except for a few rare families, it does not appear that Parkinson's disease is inherited in any simple way, although there is some tendency for it to run in families. A certain

susceptibility may be inherited but there is virtually no risk that you will pass on the disease directly to your children. (See Chapter 2.)

• *I have drunk heavily all my life, and attempted to kill myself several years ago. Is the Parkinson's disease a result of my lifestyle?*
Parkinson's disease is not the result of smoking or drinking heavily, nor is it caused by overdose of drugs (see Chapter 4). But there is one exception to this statement: drug abusers in California have been found to develop a condition indistinguishable from Parkinson's disease, caused by poisoning from the drug MPTP (see Chapter 4). In general, though, nothing that you have done during your life has increased your risk of getting Parkinson's disease.

Symptoms and physical problems

• *Do the symptoms of Parkinson's disease fluctuate through the course of the day, or do they tend to be constant from morning to night?*
Many patients with Parkinson's disease notice that their symptoms are worse at certain times of the day. This is a part of the disease. In addition, some people notice effects related to the timing of the treatment, so that they experience a particular benefit soon after taking their tablets. People who have had the disease for several years are more prone to fluctuation of symptoms throughout the day, and sometimes these changes are not obviously related to the timing of treatment. (See Chapter 8.)

• *Does Parkinson's disease affect your eyes?*
Parkinson's disease can produce certain problems with vision, although not usually severely (see Chapter 7). Blurring of vision is more commonly a side-effect of drugs, notably the anticholinergic drugs such as benzhexol (Artane) – see Chapter 8.

• *Does Parkinson's disease produce swelling of the legs and ankles?*
Ankle swelling is common if you have difficulty in getting about; this is because fluid that should be pumped out of your legs when you walk about instead collects around your ankles.

In addition, the drug amantadine and some of the dopamine agonists may provoke swelling of the ankles. One way to deal with this is to support the legs on a stool or chair when you are sitting.

- *Does Parkinson's disease affect swallowing? Is it because of the dryness of the mouth?*

Parkinson's disease can interfere with swallowing (see Chapter 7); this problem may cause some drooling of saliva from the mouth. However, dryness of the mouth and stickiness of saliva are more usually a side-effect of treatment, particularly of the anticholinergic drugs such as benzhexol (Artane) – see Chapter 8.

- *Does Parkinson's disease affect your sexual appetite or your ability to have sex?*

Difficulty in the physical aspects of a normal sexual relationship can be a major problem for people with Parkinson's disease. It may be possible to help these physical aspects of the problem by an adjustment in dosage of treatment or by adopting different positions and techniques. Professional sex counsellors are available to advise on this; you should try not to be too embarrassed to discuss the problem – it is very common, and can often be helped.

Furthermore, some of the drugs used in Parkinson's disease can interfere with sexual potency. The anticholinergic drugs, for example, may produce impotence in men, while drugs that produce sedation or confusion as side-effects will reduce sexual appetite. Rarely, sexual appetite can be enhanced dramatically by levodopa treatment, but this is a very rare side-effect. Depression also reduces sexual appetite and may be helped by antidepressant drugs (see Chapter 6).

- *Is dementia a feature of Parkinson's disease, either as a part of the disorder or as a side-effect of drugs?*

Dementia is a feature of Parkinson's disease. It is also common in the elderly population without Parkinson's disease, but the elderly patient with Parkinson's disease is more prone to it. Milder degrees of memory loss are quite common, but these are not usually troublesome, beyond a certain absent-mindedness. Some drugs, such as the anticholinergics, make memory worse, whilst other drugs used in Parkinson's disease, such as levodopa and the dopamine agonists, may produce frank confusion and hallucinations. These side-effects can occur with or without underlying dementia, although they are rather more common if there is underlying dementia. (See Chapter 6.)

- *I have constant writhing movements of my mouth and jaw, which make it difficult to eat and to keep in my false teeth. What causes this?*

These writhing movements are a form of dyskinesia (see Chapter 5). They are more usually caused by the drug treatment than the Parkinson's disease, and can be helped by modification of dosage.

- *Does Parkinson's disease cause indigestion, constipation and loss of weight?*

Parkinson's disease can produce loss of weight. Constipation can be caused by Parkinson's disease or some of the treatments. Indigestion is most commonly due to the drug treatments, particularly levodopa or bromocriptine. (See Chapters 7 and 8.)

- *I suffer from cramps at night, and can hardly walk in the morning because my foot curls inwards. What can be done about this?*

Cramps are often associated with rigidity and akinesia. Cramps are common at night in everybody, but in Parkinson's disease they are more common because the drug treatment has begun to wear off. The distortion of the foot in the morning is a rare problem, called early morning dystonia. These problems can be helped by a dose of drugs during the night, a dopamine agonist last thing at night, baclofen, or an alteration in drug dosage. (See Chapters 5 and 8.)

- *I have problems turning over in bed at night. How can this be helped?*

This problem is also due to the wearing off of drugs during the night. It can be helped in a similar way to that of night-time cramps described in the previous question. Silk sheets also help turning ability.

- *Why do I feel so depressed, even though the tablets are helping my symptoms?*

Depression is common in Parkinson's disease, and has a variety of causes. It can be helped in various ways, some by taking tablets and others not. (See Chapters 6 and 8.)

- *I have no energy or will to do anything, and my doctor says I am depressed but I do not feel miserable. How can this be so?*

Tiredness is a common symptom of Parkinson's disease, with or without depression. Depression is also common, and makes the feelings of tiredness much greater. Depression can occur without any feelings of misery, and many people who improve on antidepressant drugs were never aware that they were depressed before treatment. (See Chapter 6.)

Treatment

- *I benefit greatly from the use of levodopa, but its main drawback is the indigestion and sickness. Is there some medicine that would help this?*

The nausea and sickness of levodopa can be helped a great deal by domperidone (Motilium). Unlike some other drugs used to treat sickness, this preparation does not seem to interfere with the beneficial effects of the treatment of Parkinson's disease.

- *Can the treatment of Parkinson's disease make you confused, even if it helps you to get about more easily?*

Memory loss and confusion are side-effects of most of the treatments for Parkinson's disease, particularly in the elderly. (See Chapters 6 and 8.)

- *Will the treatment stop me getting any worse?*

The treatment will ease your symptoms considerably. It will probably not stop the condition getting worse but it can be controlled by adjusting the dose, or the type, of treatment (see Chapter 8). There is some evidence that selegiline may delay progress of the disease, but this is uncertain.

- *Is there any alternative to tablet taking?*

Taking medication is the best treatment, although it is not a cure that will take away the disease completely. You have no absolute need to take the treatment. Rarely, surgical operations can be used. Alternative medicine such as acupuncture, hypnosis and yoga can help certain symptoms but not the main problems of the disease. (See Chapters 8 and 9.)

- *Can I have an operation to cure my Parkinson's disease?*

Over recent years there have been some attempts to help or cure Parkinson's disease by surgery. These operations are usually done to people with severe problems that cannot be helped by medication. This is discussed further in Chapter 9.

- *Does the effect of the anti-Parkinsonian drugs wear off over time so that the dose needs to be progressively increased?*

Parkinson's disease tends to be a progressive condition because the loss of dopamine from the basal ganglia continues over many years. Thus, without treatment, the condition tends to become progressively worse. Current drug treatments can largely reverse the effects of loss of dopamine, but the dose of drugs will depend upon the extent to which the dopamine has been lost. Over the years it therefore tends to be necessary to make a gradual increase in the dose of drugs in order to maintain the same level of function. The speed with which the condition worsens does, however, vary substantially from person to person; some people seem to have mild disease, which continues with little change over many years.

- *Can anything be done to prevent the progression of the disease?*

Evidence from America has suggested that use of the drug selegiline (Deprenyl) early in the disease may postpone the need to begin treatment with stronger drugs, such as levodopa. This has been interpreted as indicating that the drug acts by preventing the progression of the disease. However, there are other interpretations. At the time of writing the role of selegiline in preventing disease progression remains unproven. If it does slow down progression of the condition, it may do so only in the first few years.

- *Will the drugs used for the treatment of Parkinson's disease affect pregnancy or breastfeeding?*

It is always better not to take drugs in pregnancy if these can be avoided. However, the anti-Parkinsonian drugs are not known to have any damaging effect on the unborn baby. Certainly, if you have anything more than mild Parkinson's disease, you should not discontinue your drugs; the deterioration in your Parkinson's disease would itself have a damaging effect on the pregnancy so that, for example, you may deliver prematurely or have problems in labour caused by incoordination of the muscles. If you are planning pregnancy, you should discuss this in advance with your doctor. If it is your husband who has the Parkinson's disease, the treatment that he is taking will have no effect on the baby or the pregnancy. Bromocriptine and other dopaminergic agonists (see Chapter 8) will switch off breast-feeding, so should not be used if you intend to breastfeed your baby.

Lifestyle

• *Should patients with Parkinson's disease avoid exercise or, conversely, take exercise regularly?*
It is a good idea for the patient with Parkinson's disease to take regular exercise because this will loosen the joints and help the circulation, breathing and bowel action. A schedule of regular safe exercises can be provided by physiotherapists or obtained from the Parkinson's Disease Society. However, although regular exercise is useful, you should be careful not to over-exert yourself as this will strain your muscles. Moreover, you should remember that your balance might not be good, so be careful that you do not fall or injure yourself in other ways whilst exercising. (See Chapter 9.)

• *Can I drink and smoke while taking tablets?*
Alcohol in moderate doses will not affect your treatment, although it may increase your dizziness and make you more liable to lose balance. Smoking will not interfere with your treatment, but it is bad for your health, whether or not you have Parkinson's disease.

• *Will a change of diet help me?*
Occasionally this can be helpful, but usually not – see Chapter 9.

• *Will Parkinson's disease affect my driving?*
People with Parkinson's disease are required to inform the Licensing Centre in Swansea when the diagnosis has been made because it can interfere with the ability to drive. But the Vehicle Licensing Centre will only be interested in whether the symp-toms of the condition are sufficient to interfere with driving in your particular case. With mild forms of the disorder driving is no problem and you will be allowed to continue. However, you may be issued with a licence limited to one, two or three years, after which your condition would be reassessed. The Licensing Centre usually takes advice from the doctor who knows you; he

will send his report to the Licensing Centre at their request. You would only be prevented from driving if your physical disability were such that it interfered with your ability to drive. In fact, most people are as aware of their difficulties as is their doctor. When assessing your ability to drive the Licensing Centre will take account of the side-effects of drugs, as well as the physical limitations produced by the disease; so, for example, severe dizziness would be a bar to driving.

- *Are there any drugs I should avoid?*

Some drugs do make Parkinson's disease worse, and some drugs can even produce a condition very much like Parkinson's disease in people who previously had no features of the condition. The major problems are caused by drugs used in the treatment of mental disorders, such as chlorpromazine (Largactil). However, some other important drugs are more frequently prescribed, particularly for the treatment of dizziness, such as prochlorperazine (Stemetil). Unfortunately, patients with Parkinson's disease may find that they have these drugs prescribed for them because dizziness is a common symptom of the disease. They should be avoided, if possible. (These drugs are discussed further in Chapter 1.) The antibiotic erythromycin and the sickness drug metoclopramide (Maxolon) may increase the levels of bromocriptine in the blood and provoke side effects when they are taken with bromocriptine. Pyridoxine (vitamin B6) is a vitamin currently in popular use for a variety of complaints, including premenstrual tension; pyridoxine may interfere with the action of levodopa, so reducing its effect. The effect of these latter drugs on Parkinson's disease is usually temporary, so that the effect disappears when the drug is stopped.

Other problems

- *If you have Parkinson's disease are you more prone to epilepsy, strokes or heart attacks?*

Parkinson's disease in itself does not increase the risk of epilepsy, strokes, heart attacks or brain tumours. You may know somebody who has a mixture of these diseases, but usually this is pure coincidence, brought about simply because all the diseases are common. Sometimes, a condition resembling Parkinson's disease can be produced by stroke, and strokes may give you epilepsy. These conditions can, however, be distinguished from true Parkinson's disease (see Chapter 1). Very rarely, some of the medicines used to treat Parkinson's disease can make an existing heart condition worse.

You should not confuse Parkinson's disease with other neurological conditions, such as multiple sclerosis, muscular dystrophy or motor neurone disease, of which you may have heard. These conditions are entirely different.

- *I have to have an operation that requires a general anaesthetic. Will this affect my Parkinson's disease, and what will happen if I stop my tablets for several days?*

You must be sure that your surgeon and anaesthetist are well aware that you have Parkinson's disease. Depending upon the severity of the operation, it is likely that the symptoms of your Parkinson's disease will worsen during the period of recovery after your operation. The ward staff will be aware of this, and will ensure that you are given adequate nutrition and that you receive regular physiotherapy to give you exercise. Adequate nutrition can always be given by other means, even if you are unable to swallow. The anaesthetic will not have any long-term effect on your condition. Your drug treatment will be continued throughout your hospital stay, if this is possible; even if you are not able to swallow, some treatments can be given through a tube into the stomach. If necessary, and you have severe disease, the drugs can be given through a drip into a vein of your arm. People with milder forms of Parkinson's disease are able to stop their treatment for the period of the operation without any ill effects; failure to take your tablets for these few days will not interfere with the benefit when you begin taking them again. However, stopping treatment in this way should only be done under the supervision of a doctor – do not stop the tablets of your own accord.

11

Where to get help
by the Parkinson's Disease Society

'I found it's been a great help to share my experiences with other people with Parkinson's disease. This is something that's a bit of a surprise. When you think about it, large numbers of people must go through Parkinson's disease, at least in the early stages, in sheer isolation, because they are scared and ashamed to go out and admit it to other people – they don't know anyone who has it perhaps ... I found joining the Parkinson's Disease Society brought me into contact with people. We had a weekend in a hotel where there were perhaps 50–100 people with Parkinson's disease. That alone is quite a thought. Where else do you find four dozen people with Parkinson's disease, ... all quite unabashed and all unembarrassed about it, because they know that they are with people that understand what they are doing.'

Brian Barry, person with Parkinson's disease

The Parkinson's Disease Society (PDS) receives many letters, phone calls and personal visits from people whose lives are affected by Parkinson's disease. They want to understand what is happening to them and how it will affect their future, so that they can make informed choices about their lives. Perhaps most importantly, people need encouragement to move forward from the diagnosis to being able to lead a full and active life, despite Parkinson's disease. Although, at present, there is no cure for Parkinson's disease, the increasing range of treatments available to treat the condition means that many people live full and independent lives for many years despite having Parkinson's disease.

If you, a member of your family or a friend have Parkinson's disease, knowing where to get information and advice is vital. Understanding what Parkinson's is, how it is diagnosed, what treatments are available, and who can help with any problems that arise, will help you and your family/friends maintain the best possible quality of life whilst living with Parkinson's disease. One of the main sources of such information and advice is the Parkinson's Disease Society.

The Parkinson's Disease Society of the United Kingdom was founded in 1969 by a carer, Mali Jenkins O.B.E. (1904–1989), whose sister Sarah had Parkinson's disease. The aims of the Society today are the same as they were when the Society was formed:

- To help patients and their relatives with the problems arising from Parkinson's disease.
- To collect and disseminate information on Parkinson's disease.
- To encourage and provide funds for research into Parkinson's disease.

The PDS's services are aimed at the whole 'Parkinson's family', all people who have Parkinson's disease **and** their carers, families and friends.

Welfare services

The Society runs a confidential Helpline service, which you can call Monday to Friday, 9.30am – 5.30pm. The Helpline is managed by the PDS's Welfare Counsellor, and staffed by a team of experienced and understanding volunteers. They offer a 'listening ear' for emotional issues as well as some practical advice related to Parkinson's disease.

When necessary they can refer you to PDS staff or other organisations who may be able to help you. The Helpline deals with around 4,000 calls each year, and is available on 0808 800 0303.

The PDS also provides advice on practical issues related to Parkinson's disease, including equipment, benefits, insurance, driving, financial assistance and employment. This advice, like the Helpline, is available to all people who live with Parkinson's disease, including carers, families and friends.

The PDS runs holidays at locations throughout the UK. The holidays are designed for people with Parkinson's disease, and cater for any special needs that people may have.

Respite care and residential and nursing home care can be very important for people with Parkinson's disease. The Society is involved in developing high standards of practice in all these areas, and can refer you to appropriate schemes in your area.

Publications, information and public relations

The Society publishes a wide range of publications to help people with Parkinson's disease, their families and friends, and the professionals who care for them. These include booklets and leaflets on a whole range of subjects relating to Parkinson's disease, including the treatments available, physiotherapy, speech and language therapy, occupational therapy, clothing, and sex. A video, aimed specifically at people who are newly diagnosed and their families, is also available.

If you become a member of the PDS you will receive a copy of *The Parkinson*, the Society's membership newsletter, four times a year. *The Parkinson* is the PDS's flagship publication, and includes information on living with Parkinson's disease, the latest advances in research, and details of the Society's activities.

The PDS's Information Department will deal with your queries on all aspects of Parkinson's disease, including treatment. This may involve providing information not included in PDS publications, which may have to be obtained from alternative sources. If necessary the Information Department will refer you to another organization or agency to help you get the information you need.

Raising awareness of Parkinson's disease and the PDS is also a major part of the Society's activities. Using the media, advertising, and information materials, the PDS is determined to improve the understanding of Parkinson's disease among the general public. The Society is recognized as the national voice of people with Parkinson's. Many people with Parkinson's disease experience unfair prejudice, often as a result of ignorance. The PDS is campaigning to end unfair discrimination and improve the standard of care offered to people with Parkinson's disease.

Research

The Parkinson's Disease Society spends more than £1.5 million annually on medical and welfare research projects. The Research Department organizes research conferences and open days for Parkinson's Disease Society members and health and social care professionals.

The Parkinson's Disease Society funds the Brain Research Centre, the only resource of its kind in the UK, where donated brain from both people with, and without Parkinson's, are studied.

To find out more about Parkinson's Disease Society-funded research call 020 7932 1346 or
e-male: research@parkinsons.org.uk

Special Parkinson's Research Interest Group (SPRING) is a special interest group of the Parkinson's Disease Society that focuses upon medical research.

Contact SPRING on 01483 281307
or e-mail spring@parkinsons.org.uk

Local branches

As Brian Barry's quote at the beginning of this chapter testifies, meeting other people living with Parkinson's disease to share experiences and provide mutual support can be very helpful. The Society has over 200 local branches throughout the UK, all run entirely by volunteers, usually people with Parkinson's disease and their families. PDS branches offer help, advice and mutual support. They usually meet on a monthly basis, and can provide practical advice on local facilities and the work of the Society. Many branches have Welfare Visitors who may visit you in your home.

Branches also organize a variety of social activities for members, some of which raise awareness and funds.

Service Provision for People with Parkinson's Disease and their Carers

Help required	Provided by	Who to contact
Home help/care services	Home care service	Home care organizer at local authority social services
Meals on Wheels	Meals on Wheels service	Local social services department
Help with bathing	District nurse (practical help), Occupational therapist (advice on equipment)	Your GP, Occupational therapy dept. at your local social services
Laundry service	District health authority or local social services	District nurse or local social services department
Advice on washing, dressing and daily tasks	Occupational therapist	Occupational therapy dept. at your local social services
Advice on dealing with incontinence	District nurse or continence adviser	Your GP, Continence Foundation

Aids and adaptations to improve living at home	Occupational therapist	Occupational therapy dept. at your local social services, Disabled Living Foundation (advice)
Communication aids	Speech and language therapist	District speech and language therapist at local hospital, GP
Advice on special equipment and where to obtain it	Occupational therapist, Disabled Living Foundation, or through district nurse	Occupational therapy dept. at your local social services, Disabled Living Foundation, GP
Short-term hire of equipment	Local social services, British Red Cross	Local social services, British Red Cross
Speech and swallowing problems	Speech and language therapist	District speech and language therapist at local hospital, GP
Sitters, minders, care attendants	Local social services, voluntary agencies such as Age Concern	Local social services, voluntary organizations, Yellow Pages
Day centre care	Local social services, local health authority, voluntary agencies	Local social service, local health authority, voluntary agencies

Help required	Provided by	Who to contact
Short-term (respite) care	Local social services, voluntary agencies	Local social services, voluntary agencies, PDS (for advice)
Advice on holidays	Holiday Care Service, PDS	Holiday Care Service, PDS
Residential/nursing care homes	Local authority and privately owned registered homes	Local social services department will have a list, PDS (for advice)
Mutual support groups for carers	Carers National Association, Crossroads Care	Carers National Association, Crossroads Care
Advice on all matters	Citizen's Advice Bureau, PDS	Citizen's Advice Bureau, PDS
Benefits, income maintenance, income support, housing benefit, council tax, etc.	Local Department of Social Security, Housing benefit department, Citizen's Advice Bureau	Local Department of Social Security, local authority housing department, Citizen's Advice Bureau
Help with paying for residential care	Local Department of Social Security	Local Department of Social Security, PDS (for advice)

Help with driving and other mobility needs	Orange badge scheme, Motability, Mobility Allowance, Drivers/Mobility Assessment Centres	Local social services, Local Department of Social Security, Drivers/Mobility Assessment Centres, PDS (for advice), Disabled Living Foundation
Travelling assistance	Tripscope, local transport schemes such as Dial-a-Ride, St John's Ambulance, British Red Cross	Tripscope, Citizen's Advice Bureau, local library, St John's Ambulance, British Red Cross
Help with costs of travel	Various concessionary bus and rail schemes	British Rail, local bus operators
Help with prescriptions, optical and dental treatment and fares to hospital	Local Department of Social Security, Citizen's Advice Bureau	Local Department of Social Security, Citizen's Advice Bureau
Help with paying for holidays and intermittent needs, shortfall in nursing homes	Local social services, Benevolent and charitable institutions	Charities Digest (available in local reference library), PDS (for advice and help in making application)

YAPP&RS (Young Alert Parkinsonians Partners and Relatives)

The Young Alert Parkinsonians Partners and Relatives (YAPP&RS) is the PDS's group for younger people with Parkinson's disease – people of working age. The YAPP&RS have their own magazine, meetings, library service and computer link and, like the Society itself, cater for carers, families and friends.

Field services

The PDS has staff based throughout the UK, divided into three regions, north, central and south. They liaise with local health care providers and PDS branches and promote the Society's work. Some of the field staff are involved in providing training for health and social care professionals. In 1995 the Scottish Resource, an office based in Glasgow, was opened. This is the PDS's first office away from its main headquarters in London.

Fundraising

The PDS could not function without money. The Fundraising Department works extremely hard to raise money to fund all the Society's activities. Activities include events, a prize draw, links with major companies and a legacy campaign.

If you would like to become a member of the PDS or you would like further information or advice on anything relating to Parkinson's disease or the work of the Society, please contact us at the following address:

Parkinson's Disease Society of the United Kingdom
215 Vauxhall Bridge Road
London SW1V 1EJ
Telephone: 020 7931 8080 Helpline: 0808 800 0303
(Monday–Friday 9.30 am – 5.30 pm)
Email: enquiries@parkinsons.org.uk
www.parkinsons.org.uk

Glossary

acetylcholine One of the chemicals involved in passing messages through the brain in order to coordinate movement. Some of the drugs used in Parkinson's disease affect the action of this chemical.
adrenal A gland that is situated just above the kidneys. The adrenal gland is one of the tissues that have been implanted into the basal ganglia as an attempted surgical cure for Parkinson's disease.
agonist A synthetic drug that mimics the action of one of the naturally occurring brain chemicals (neurotransmitters). For example, dopamine agonist drugs are used in Parkinson's disease to bypass the deficiency of dopamine.
akinesia Slowness in the initiations of movement; similar to bradykinesia. A cardinal sign of Parkinson's disease.
amantadine A drug which was first used to treat virus infections but which is now used as a second-line treatment for Parkinson's disease.
antagonist A drug which prevents the action of a naturally occurring chemical within the nervous system. For example, anticholinergic drugs block the action of acetylcholine and thereby compensate for the deficiency of dopamine.
anticholinergic A class of drugs, such as benzhexol, used in the treatment of Parkinson's disease. These drugs work by blocking the action of acetylcholine, one of the brain chemicals involved in transmitting messages within the brain.
apomorphine One of the class of dopamine agonist drugs, used for the treatment of Parkinson's disease. Apomorphine is used only for the treatment of on-off syndrome and has to be given by injection under the skin (subcutaneous).
apraxia Loss of ability to carry out skilled movements. In Parkinson's disease, the term is usually used for 'apraxia of lid-opening', or difficulty in holding the eyes open.
arteriosclerosis Deposition of material on the inside of the arteries which leads to narrowing of their calibre and reduced supply of blood.

autonomic nervous system Part of the nervous system that controls heart rate, blood pressure, functions of the bladder, and bowel and sexual capacity.

baclofen A drug to prevent muscle spasm which is sometimes useful in Parkinson's disease for treating night-time cramps and dystonias.

basal ganglia Part of the nervous system that co-ordinates movement. The main site of damage in Parkinson's disease.

benzhexol One of the group of anticholinergic drugs used for the treatment of Parkinson's disease.

benztropine One of the group of anticholinergic drugs used for the treatment of Parkinson's disease.

blepharospasm Involuntary contraction of the muscles around the eyes so that the eyes close in spasm for seconds or minutes at a time. A form of dystonia. Not usually seen in Parkinson's disease but in conditions that resemble it.

bradykinesia Slowness of movement. Similar to akinesia.

bradyphrenia A term used to describe slowness of thinking (but without loss of memory) said to be a feature of some patients with Parkinson's disease.

bromocriptine One of a class of drugs known as dopamine agonists, or dopaminergic drugs, used to treat Parkinson's disease.

chorea Involuntary movement, manifest as twitching, fidgeting or writhing movements. The commonest form of dyskinesia.

domperidone A drug used to prevent nausea and vomiting, common side-effects of the main drugs used in the treatment of Parkinson's disease.

dopamine One of the brain chemicals involved in transmitting messages from one nerve cell to another (neurotransmitter). Loss of dopamine from the basal ganglia is the major cause of the symptoms and signs of Parkinson's disease.

dopaminergic drug A synthetic drug that mimics the action of dopamine in the brain and so bypasses the dopamine deficiency in Parkinson's disease.

dyskinesia Twitching, fidgety, writhing or flapping movements that occur usually as a side-effect of levodopa treatment. Distinct from tremor.

dystonia An involuntary sustained contraction of one set of muscles, similar to a spasm, which may persist for several minutes. Often affects the foot in Parkinson's disease.

encephalitis lethargica A viral infection of the brain which was often followed years later by a form of Parkinson's disease; now virtually disappeared.

end-of-dose deterioration One of the problems of long-standing Parkinson's disease in which the effects of each dose of drug do not last until the next dose is due.

festinating Refers to the gait of Parkinson's disease in which the person makes a series of rapid short steps, often when approaching objects or narrow openings, such as doorways. It is often associated with imbalance.

freezing Describes the sudden, unpredictable akinesia that usually comes on during walking and causes complete inability to move.

hypotension Fall in blood pressure. In Parkinson's disease, often caused by levodopa-containing drugs or sometimes by autonomic failure.

idiopathic Cause unknown. 'Ordinary' Parkinson's disease is often known as idiopathic Parkinson's disease and distinguished from Parkinsonism.

Lewy body A change within the nerve cells of the Parkinsonian brain. When viewed under the microscope, the Lewy body appears as a spherical 'object' within the damaged nerve cells of the substantia nigra.

lysuride One of the class of dopamine agonist, or dopaminergic, drugs used for the treatment of Parkinson's disease.

Madopar One of the main drugs used for the treatment of Parkinson's disease. Madopar consists of a combination of levodopa and another drug to block some of its side-effects.

methixene One of the group of anticholinergic drugs used for the treatment of Parkinson's disease.

micrographia The difficulty in writing that occurs in Parkinson's disease. Typically, the writing starts at normal size and becomes progressively smaller as writing continues.

MPTP A poisonous substance which damages the nerve cells of the substantia nigra and produces a condition virtually indistinguishable from Parkinson's disease.

neurotransmitter A chemical substance that is important for the transmission of messages from one nerve cell to the next; e.g. dopamine, acetylcholine and noradrenaline.

noradrenaline One of the brain neurotransmitters involved in passing messages from one nerve cell to the next.

on-off A complication, usually of long-standing Parkinson's disease, in which the patient experiences rapid swings from mobility to immobility several times each day.

orphenadrine One of the group of anticholinergic drugs used for the treatment of Parkinson's disease.

pallidotomy A form of stereotactic surgery (see below). This is a new treatment, under investigation, which may help akinesia, rigidity and dyskinesia.

paralysis agitans Another term for Parkinson's disease.

Parkinsonism A term used for diseases that resemble Parkinson's disease but are caused by quite different changes within the brain.

Penject A method of giving apomorphine by injection. The Penject is a syringe which can be clipped inside the pocket, like a fountain pen.

pergolide One of the group of dopamine agonist, or dopaminergic, drugs used for the treatment of Parkinson's disease.

procyclidine One of the group of anticholinergic drugs used for the treatment of Parkinson's disease.

rigidity Stiffness of the muscles; one of the main signs of Parkinson's disease.

selegiline A drug used in Parkinson's disease to prolong the action of levodopa and which may delay the progression of the disease.

Sinemet One of the main drugs used for the treatment of Parkinson's disease. Sinemet consists of a combination of levodopa and another drug to block some of its side-effects.

stereotactic surgery A form of surgery in which a small area of destruction is made within the basal ganglia to treat tremor and sometimes dyskinesia.

subcutaneous An injection under the skin. The main route for the administration of apomorphine.

substantia nigra Part of the basal ganglia, within the brain, involved in co-ordinating movement. The major change in the brain of Parkinson's disease is loss of dopamine-containing cells from the substantia nigra.

syndrome A term used to describe conditions which may have more than one cause but which present with similar features, e.g. Parkinsonism.

titubation Involuntary tremor of the head.

tone, muscle tone The slight stiffness that is present in the muscles even when they are perfectly relaxed. In Parkinson's disease the tone is increased.

tremor Involuntary shaking of the limbs and head. (Tremor is common but not universal in Parkinson's disease and also occurs in other conditions, such as benign essential tremor.)

yo-yo-ing A severe form of on-off syndrome in which the patient undergoes swings in mobility often from severe rigidity and akinesia to florid dyskinesia.

Useful Addresses and Websites

United Kingdom

Parkinson's Disease Society
215 Vauxhall Bridge Road, London SW1V 1EJ
Tel: 020 7931 8080
www.parkinsons.org.uk

Age Concern

www.ageconcern.org.uk
ENGLAND: Astral House, 1268 London Road, London SW16 4ER
Tel: 020 8765 7200
Offers support for older people and those who care for them. Local groups provide services such as day centres, lunch clubs and transport visiting schemes. They also publish 'Fact Sheets' offering advice and information.

SCOTLAND: 113 Rose Street, Edinburgh EH3 3DT
Tel: 0131 220 3345

WALES: 4th Floor, 1 Cathedral Road, Cardiff CF1 9SD
Tel: 029 2037 1566

Association of Crossroads Care Attendant Schemes
10 Regent Place, Rugby, Warwickshire CV21 2PN
Tel: 01788 565498
Provides care attendants who come into the home to give the carer a break. 180 autonomous schemes throughout England, Scotland and Wales. 10 regional offices including:

WALES: Watton Chambers, the Watton, Brecon
Tel: 01874 623090
www.crossroads.org.uk

Crossroads Scotland Care Attendant Schemes
24 George Square, Glasgow G2 1EG
Tel: 0141 226 3793
www.neuroconsult.co.uk
This website, founded by Professor Sagar, provides comprehensive
information on neurological disorders, including Parkinson's disease.
Separate, but similar, organization for Scotland.

British Association For Counselling
1 Regent Place, Rugby, Warwickshire CV21 2PJ
Tel: 01788 550899
Provides list of counsellors divided into counties, giving counsellors'
qualifications, type of problems counselled and probable cost, and
information sheet with counselling guidelines.
www.bac.co.uk

British Red Cross Society

ENGLAND: 9 Grosvenor Crescent, London SW1X 7EJ
Tel: 020 7235 5454

SCOTLAND: 204 Bath Street, Glasgow G2 4HL
Tel: 0141 332 9591

Provides equipment, transport and courses in first aid.
www.redcross.org.uk

Carers National Association

NATIONAL: 20/25 Glasshouse Yard, London EC1A 4JT
Tel: 020 7490 8818
Helpline: 0808 8087777
Information and support to people who are caring at home.
Branches and local offices throughout the UK, including:

SCOTLAND: 11 Queens Crescent, Glasgow G4 9AF
Tel: 0141 353 2726

NORTHERN IRELAND: 11 Lower Crescent, Belfast BT7 1NR
Tel: 028 9043 9843
www.carersni.org

Charity Commission
Harnsworth House, 13–15 Bouverie Street, London EC4Y 8DP
Tel: 0870 333 0123
A government department responsible for regulating and
investigating, where necessary, the activities of charities.
www.charity-commission.gov.uk

Community Health Council (*in England and Wales*)
Local Health Council (*in Scotland*)
Look in the phone book or in Yellow Pages under 'Consumer and Trading Standards Organizations'. Information and advice on anything to do with the health services.

The Continence Foundation
307 Hatton Square, 16 Baldwin Gardens, London EC1N 7RJ
Tel: 020 74046875
Helpline: 020 7831 9831
An organization which provides information and education on continence for professionals and the general public. A Continence Information Helpline is staffed by continence advisors Monday to Friday from 9.30 – 4.30 pm.
www.continence-foundation.org.uk

Counsel and Care
Lower Ground Floor, Twyman House, 16 Bonny Street, London NW1 9PG
Tel: 020 7485 1550
Advice service for elderly people, their relatives and professionals; information and leaflets; grants to help people to remain in or return to their homes.
www.counselandcare.org.uk

Cruse – Bereavement Care
Helpline: 0870 1671677
ENGLAND: Cruse House, 126 Sheen Road, Richmond, Surrey TW9 1UR
Tel: 020 89399530
SCOTLAND: 18 South Trinity Road, Edinburgh EH5 3PN
Tel: 0131 551 1511

Offers support and counselling to anyone who has been bereaved.

Department for Work and Pensions
Richmond House, 79 Whitehall, London SW1A 2NL
Tel: 020 7238 0800
Government department responsible for social security issues.
www.dwp.gov.uk

Department of Health, Social Services and Public Safety (*Northern Ireland*)
Information Office, Castle Buildings, Stormont, Belfast BT4 3SJ

Tel: 028 905 20500
www.dhsspsni.gov.uk

Disabled Living Foundation
380–384 Harrow Road, London W9 2HU
Tel: 020 7289 6111
Provides advice and information on all sorts of aids and equipment
for people with disabilities.

Health Information Service
Freephone 0800 665544
A national freephone Health Information Service providing a
helpline where people with disabilities and others with health
concerns can seek information. This service links together the
telephone helpline information services operated by the Regional
Health Authorities since April 1991. Callers dialling the 0800
number are transferred automatically to their local service.
Information on various conditions, NHS Services, waiting times,
local Patient's Charter Standards, how to complain about the NHS,
health maintenance, self-help groups and voluntary services are
provided by the helpline. The service is also available to health
professionals to enable them to answer patients' queries.
The service is generally open between 10.00 am and 5.00 pm,
although some regional information centres are
open for longer hours.

Help the Aged
207–221 Pentonville Road, London W1 9UZ
Tel: 020 7278 1114
Offers support and advice to elderly people and their families.
www.helptheaged.org.uk

Holiday Care Service
2nd Floor, Imperial Buildings, Victoria Road, Horley, Surrey
RH6 7PZ
Tel: 01293 774535
Holiday information and support for people who have difficulties
finding a holiday due to age, disability or severe financial pressures.

Local Authority (Council)
Look in the phone book under the name of your county, district,
metropolitan or borough council. If you are not sure of the name,
look in Yellow Pages under 'Local Government'. There are usually
different phone numbers for different departments, so look under
the name of the department you want to contact, or ask for the

information or enquiries department if you are not sure which department you want.

Your local authority is responsible for a whole range of services including housing and social services.

Local Transport Authority
Look in the phone book under the name of your county. Listed in some areas as a department of the county council. In other areas, listed as '. . . (County name) Passenger Transport Executive'.

Information about concessionary fares and other local authority transport schemes for people with disabilities.

National Association of Citizen's Advice Bureaux

ENGLAND: Myddleton House, 115/123 Pentonville Road, London N1 9LZ
Tel: 020 783 32181

SCOTLAND: (CITIZEN'S ADVICE SCOTLAND) 26 George Square, Edinburgh EH8 9LD
Tel: 0131 667 0156

NORTH WALES: 1 Nant Hall Road, Prestatyn, Clwyd LL19 9LR
Tel: 01745 855400

SOUTH WALES: Andrews Building (Suite 3–23), 67 Queen Street, Cardiff CF1 4UA
Tel: 01222 377 407

Advice centres with local offices.
www.nacab.org.uk

National Association of Councils for Voluntary Service (NACVS)
3rd Floor, Arundel Court, 177 Arundel Street, Sheffield S1 2NU
Tel: 0114 278 6636
An information body that can tell you about local Councils for Voluntary Service.
www.nacvs.org.uk

National Care Homes Association
45/49 Leather Care, London, EC1N 7TJ
Tel: 020 7831 7090
A federation of local associations of private homes. Offers advice on anything to do with private residential care – can put you in touch with member associations in your area.
www.ncha.gb.com

National Council for Voluntary Organisations (NCVO)
Regents Wharf, 8 All Saints Street, London N1 9RL
Tel: 020 7713 6161
Can give you information about voluntary organizations in your
area.
www.ncvo–vol.org.uk

National Listening Library
12 Lant Street, London SE1 1QH
Tel: 020 7407 9417
A subscription lending library service of talking books for people
with disabilities.
www.listening–books.org.uk

Northern Ireland Council for Voluntary Action
61 Duncairn Gardens, Belfast BT15 2GB
Tel: 028 9087 7777

Radar (Royal Association for Disability and Rehabilitation)
12 City Forum, 250 City Road, London EC1V 8AF
Telephone: 020 7250 3222
Publishes information on aids and equipment, access, holidays,
mobility, sport, leisure and campaigning.
www.radar.org.uk

Relate (National Marriage Guidance)
Herbert Gray College, Little Church Street, Rugby, Warwickshire
CV21 3AP
Tel: 01788 573241
Relationship counselling, nationally and locally.
www.relate.org.uk

Samaritans
A voluntary organization offering confidential emotional support 24
hours a day. 171 branches in England, Scotland and Wales.
Look in the telephone book for your nearest branch.
www.samaritans.org.uk

Scottish Council for Voluntary Organisations
18/19 Claremont Crescent, Edinburgh EH7 4QD
Tel: 0131 556 3882
www.scvo.org.uk

The Scottish Executive
St Andrew's House, Regent Road, Edinburgh EH1 3DG

Tel: 0131 556 8400
A government department responsible for Scottish matters.
www.scotland.gov.uk

Talking Newspapers Association of the United Kingdom
90 High Street, Heathfield, East Sussex TN21 8JD
Tel: 01435 866102
www.tnauk.org.uk

Tripscope
The Vassall Centre, Gill Avenue, Bristol BS16 2QQ
Tel: 08457 585 641
Advice on travel and transport for people with disabilities.

Wales Council for Voluntary Action
Batltic House, Mount Stuart Square, Cardiff CF10 SFH
Tel: 029 204 31700
www.wcva.org.uk

The Welsh Office
Cathays Park, Cardiff CD1 3N2
Tel: 01222 825111
A government department responsible for Welsh issues.

Winged Fellowship Trust
Angel House, 32 Pentonville Road, London N1 9XD
Tel: 020 7833 2594
Holidays and respite care for physically disabled people.
www.wft.org.uk

Useful Contacts/Addresses – Driving

Disabled Drivers Association
Ashwellthorpe, Norwich NR16 1EX
Tel: 01508 489449
www.dda.org.uk
Disabled Drivers Motor Club Ltd
Cottingham Way, Thrapston, Northants NN14 4PL
Tel: 01832 734724

Mobility Test and Assessment Centres

Cornwall Friends Mobility Centre
Tehidy House, Royal Cornwall Hospital, Truro, Cornwall TR1 3LJ
Tel: 01872 254 920

Derby Regional Disability Centre
Kingsway Hospital, Kingsway, Derby DE22 3LZ
Tel: 01332 371 929

Disability Action
2 Annadale Avenue, Belfast BT3 9EDR
Tel: 028 9029 7880

Edinburgh Driving Assessment Service
Mobility Centre, Astley Ainslie Hospital, 133 Grange Loan,
Edinburgh, EH9 2HL
Tel: 0131 537 9192

Mobility Advice & Vehicle Information Service
'D' Wing, Macadam Avenue, Old Wokingham Road, Crowthorne,
Berks RG45 6XD
Tel: 01344 661000

Mobility Centre
Hunters Moor Regional Rehabilitation Centre, Hunters Road,
Newcastle-upon-Tyne NE2 4NR
Tel: 0191 219 5694

Mobility Information Service
Unit B1 Greenwood Court, Cartmel Drive, Shrewsbury SY1 3TB
Tel: 01743 463072

Queen Elizabeth's Foundation Mobility Centre
Fountain Drive, Carhalton, Surrey SM5 4NR
Tel: 020 8770 1157

Rookwood Driving Assessment Centre
Rookwood Hospital, Fairwater Road, Llandaff, Cardiff CF5 2YN
Tel: 029 20555730

Wales Disabled Drivers Assessment Centre
18 Plas Newydd, Whitchurch, Cardiff CF4 1NR
Tel: 01222 615276

Australia

Parkinson's New South Wales Inc
Concord Hospital, Bld 64, Hospital Road, Concord, NSW 2139, Australia
www.parkinsonsnsw.org.au

Parkinson's Victoria Inc
20 Kingston Road, Cheltenham, Victoria 3192, Australia
www.parkinsons–vic.org.au

Parkinson's Western Australia Inc
PO Box 910, West Perth, WA 6872, Australia
www.cuarte.com.au/parkinsons

Belgium

Association Parkinson
Rue Champ des Alenettes, 709 fratore en Condroz, Belgium

Brazil

Associacão Brasil Parkinson
Fortaleza, ceara 60451–970, Brazil
www.parkinson.org.br

Canada

The Parkinson Foundation of Canada
4211 Yonge Street, Suite 316, Toronto, Ontario, M2P 2A9, Canada
www.parkinson.ca

Denmark

Dansk Parkinson Forening, Bomlaerkevej 12, Horsholm, 2970, Denmark

Finland

Finnish Parkinson's Association
Suomen Parkinson Gtto, Prs 905, Tunai, 20101, Finland
www.parkinson.fi

France

Association France Parkinson
37 bis Rue la Fontaine, Paris 75016, France

Germany

Deutsche Parkinson Vereinigung
Moselstrasse 31, Neuss 41464, Germany

Japan

Japan Parkinson Disease Association
2–2–8, Nishiwaseda, Shinjuku-ku, Tokyo, Japan

The Netherlands

Parkinson Patienten Vereniging
Postbus 46, 3980 CA Bunnik, The Netherlands

New Zealand

The Parkinson Society of New Zealand Inc.
PO Box 10392, Wellington, New Zealand

Norway

Norges Parkinsonforbund
Schweigaardsgt, 34, by ggf, appg.2, Oslo 0191, Norway

South Africa
South African Parkinson Association
Private Bag, 36, Bryanstan 2021, South Africa

Spain

Parkinson España
c/de la Torre, 14 bajos, 08006 Barcelona, Spain

Sweden

Svenska Parkinsonforbundet
Karlagatan 23, S-416 61 Goteborg, Sweden

Switzerland

Schweizerische Parkinsonvereinigung
Geuerbestrasse, 12 case Postace 123, 8132 EGG, Switzerland
www.parkinson.ch

United States

American Parkinson's Disease Association
1250 Hylan Boulevard, Suite 4B, Staten Island, New York
10305–1946, USA
www.apdaparkinson.com

National Parkinson Foundation
Bob Hope Parkinson Research Centre, 1501 NW Ninth Avenue,
Bob Hope Road, Miami, Florida 33136, USA
www.parkinson.org

Parkinson's Disease Foundation
William Black Medical Research Building,
710 West 168th Street, New York 10032–9982, USA
www.parkinsons-foundation.org

United Parkinson Foundation
823 West Washington Boulevard, Chicago, Illinois 60607, USA

HOW CAN I HELP?

Research into Parkinson's disease requires money for staff and equipment. One way you can help is by donating money to charities that support research into Parkinson's disease. It does not matter how small a sum this is, because most of the large sums of money are made up of many small contributions. If you cannot afford any money yourself – perhaps because you are retired or no longer able to work – then maybe you could persuade others who can afford it. The Parkinson's Disease Society, which funds a great deal of research into Parkinson's disease, has a number of local branches that are often actively engaged in fundraising; if you do not belong to one you could contact your nearest branch or the Society's head office, who would be only too willing to provide details of how you can help.

It is also possible to help without providing any money at all. Much of the research into Parkinson's disease requires volunteers to undertake tests, or to provide blood samples, that can help to identify exactly what has gone wrong – much of the information obtained in this book has been obtained from just this sort of research on volunteers. Again, the Parkinson's Disease Society is able to provide information on research projects for which you could volunteer – contact them for further information (the address is provided elsewhere in this book). You will be told well in advance of the sort of things you would be required to do, and you are always able to say no if the research does not appeal to you. Many research projects also require healthy volunteers for comparison, so perhaps you could also persuade your husband, wife or relatives to take part. Do contact the Parkinson's Disease Society if you are interested in research into Parkinson's disease.

INDEX